Naturally Delicious Meals for Baby

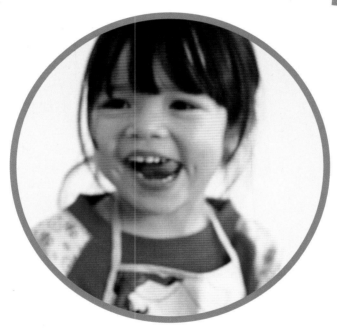

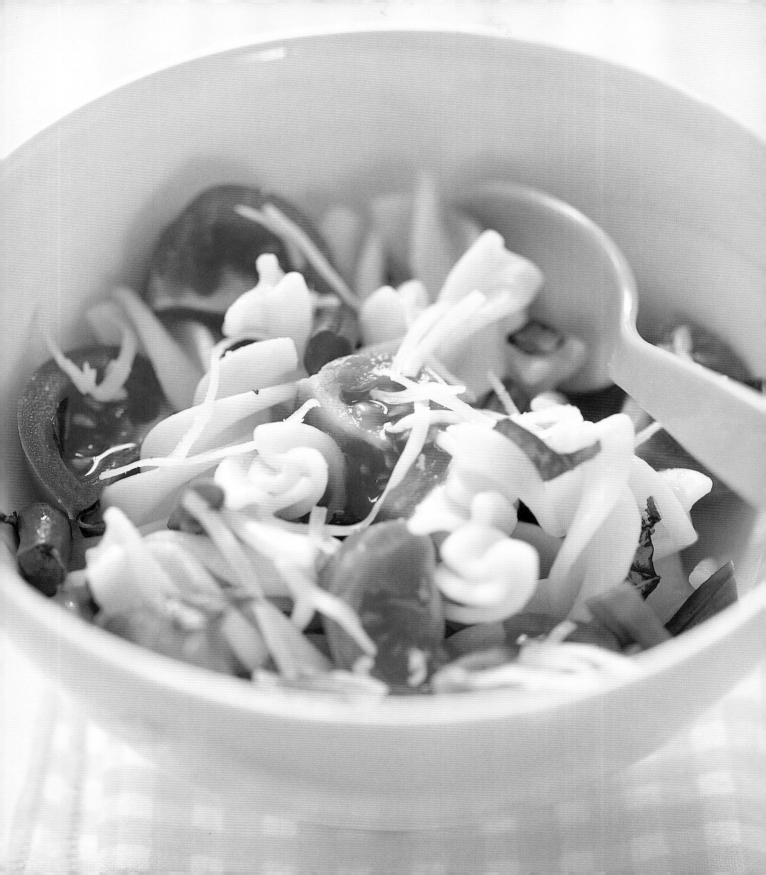

Naturally Delicious Meals for Baby

Over 150 Fun, Fresh and Easy Recipes to Nourish Your Baby and Toddler

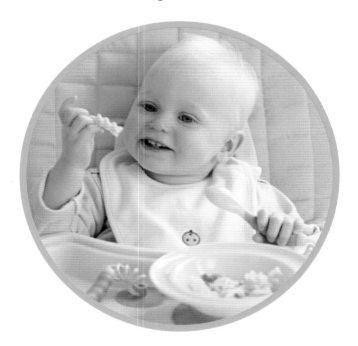

Gerrie Hawes with Bruce Hudson and Ali Hanan

Marlowe & Company
New York

For giggling Sandra, time for tennis Malcolm,
and in loving memory of my grandparents,
Daisy and Percy, Elsie and Walter.

NATURALLY DELICIOUS MEALS FOR BABY: *Over 150 Fun, Fresh, and Easy Recipes to*
Nourish Your Baby and Toddler

This book contains general advice and recipes suitable for babies and
children. If you have specific concerns, special dietary needs, or a family
history of allergies or food intolerances, you should seek the advice of
your paediatrician or other specialist medical practitioner.

Published by Marlowe & Company
An Imprint of Avalon Publishing Group Incorporated
245 West 17th Street • 11th floor
New York, NY 10011

AVALON
publishing group incorporated

Senior editor: Muna Reyal
Designer: Alison Fenton
Photographer: Sandra Lane
Stylist: Cathy Sinker
Food stylists: Krissy Schmidt,
    Jacqueline Bellefontaine and Lizzie Harris
Copy editor: Anne Newman
Editorial assistant: Cecilia Desmond
Production: Sha Huxtable and Alice Holloway

Library of Congress Control Number: 2005931783
ISBN 1-56924-312-3
10 9 8 7 6 5 4 3 2 1

Distributed by Publishers Group West
Color reproduction by Sang Choy
Printed and bound in China by C & C Offset Printing Company Ltd

Contents

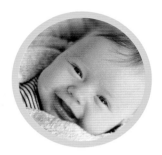

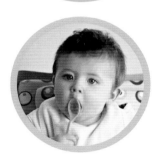

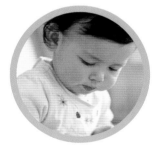

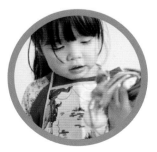

FOREWORD

Why *Naturally Delicious Meals for Baby*

Naturally Delicious Meals for Baby evolved from conversations I had with parents while working on Fresh Daisy. This is a book for real parents living in the real world. There is nothing complicated about making delicious baby food—but there are some basics you need to know before you dive in.

I start with recipes for you, not only to encourage you to think about your own relationship with food before you start teaching your child, but also because there's now evidence that babies start to develop taste preferences before the first purée passes their lips.

Naturally Delicious Meals for Baby is also for parents who look through cookbooks for babies and toddlers and say, "How the hell do they expect me to decorate baby food with eyes, ears, and toenails when I've got a screaming child scattering toys around the room?" Hey, I hear you. Hopefully you'll find my approach a refreshing change.

Developing a good relationship with food

Learning to eat well and educate the palate is as important as learning your ABC's, which is why I want to introduce your baby to the tastes and textures of *real* food. Studies by Dr. Gillian Harris at the UK's Birmingham University show that the foods you feed your baby now will have a profound effect on their health for life. If you consider that nearly a third of all children aged 6–11 in the USA are overweight, as well as the mounting evidence that behavior and brain development are affected by diet, it does raise the question: If we are what we eat, then what on earth are our children eating? What could be better than the real taste, natural color, and wholesome nutrition of fresh fruit, vegetables, meat, and fish?

Ultimately your baby should eat as you do. Besides, life's just too short to make everyone's favorite meals every night. That's one of the many reasons why we've included a section of deliciously healthy meals for you and why most of the toddler dishes are adaptable to adult tastes.

Why Fresh Daisy?

As somebody who is passionate about the taste, textures, and flavors of food, working for a major food manufacturer was a surprisingly depressing eye opener. Every time I visited the factory, it didn't matter whether it was baby food, tomato soup, pasta in sauce, or baked beans being cooked, it always had the same underlying smell. It's an odd, not completely unpleasant smell, but very different from what you'd smell in a domestic kitchen. This was when the light bulb started to flash. I was working on toddler food, and began to question why children seem to have such a taste for highly processed food. I could only assume that taste preferences develop very early on, which drew my attention to the standards of commercially available baby food.

I launched the Fresh Daisy range of baby foods in 2003—using the simple principles any parent would use if time permitted: the best organic seasonal food, sourced direct from the farmer whenever possible; steaming freshly prepared ingredients without the addition of antibrowning or other processing agents, then fast freezing in individual portions. Simple. Pure.

I began to realize that the reliance on overprocessed food was an extremely damaging way to bring up a child. My fears were confirmed when we started to do tastings at baby shows. Babies brought up on commercial jars, cans, and pots wouldn't eat our product, yet those brought up on homemade food lapped it up. Nursery owners also vented their frustration at having to "rewean" babies off sterilized baby food on to homemade food by gradually reintroducing fresh products.

I urge you to have a go at making at least one or two of the cooked purées yourself—and compare the taste, color and texture to those of most commercial baby foods. Once you've tasted frozen baby food (your own or store-bought) I think you'll find it hard to reach for the jar.

The future

Having tried to ignore my desire to revolutionize baby food for eight years, I was inspired by my now husband to give it a try, influenced by that typical pioneering spirit New Zealanders seem to foster. Fresh Daisy feels more like a vocation than a business—success is seeing the quality of baby food significantly improve and parents understanding that it really does matter what a baby eats.

So *vive la révolution*! Three years after launching I'm still battling away, trying to convince the major supermarkets to change the whole baby food sector. It's very much two steps forward and one step back, or maybe a bit more the other way around. But what hasn't changed is my passion for improving the standard of commercially available baby food.

Recipe for success?

Thanks for buying the book, enjoy the journey, experiment with tastes for you and your baby and help spread the word that fresh is best. And if you don't have time to make your own, frozen baby food may be available in your supermarket!

Gerie Hawes

Introduction

A beginner's guide on how and what to feed your baby. Everything from a nutritional guide to the right equipment to buy (and even a word about poop).

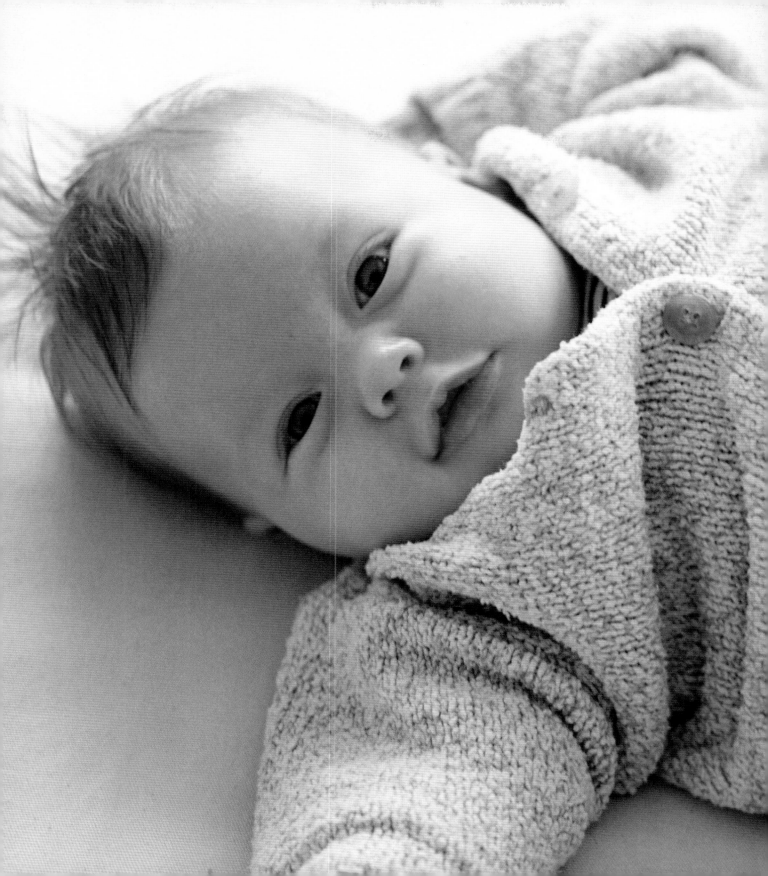

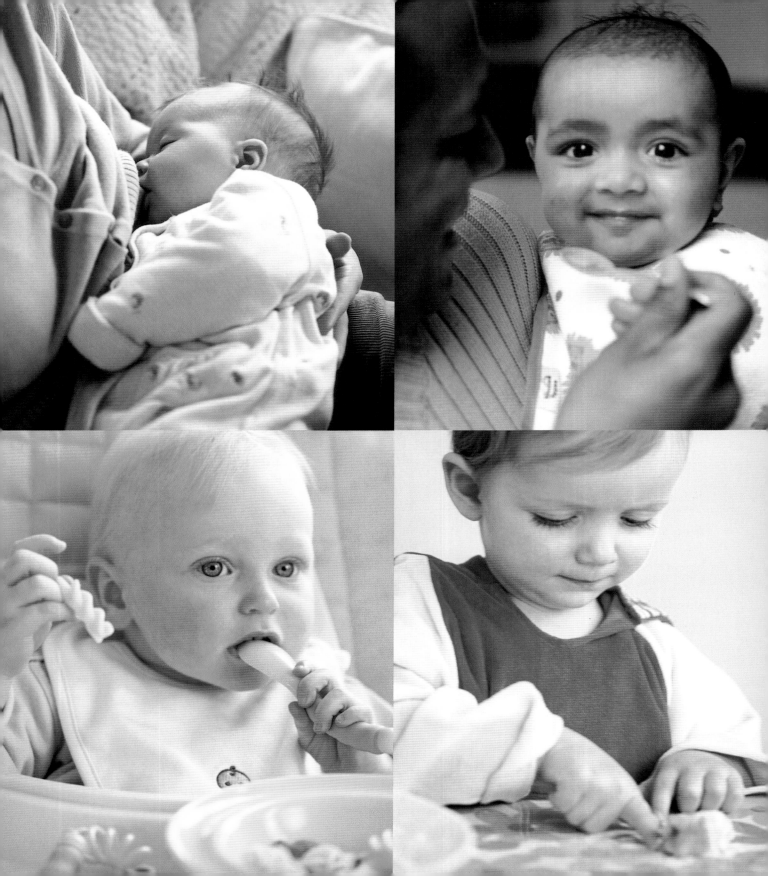

How to use this book

You come first

This book starts with you. Yes, your baby is important, but so are you. A happy parent usually means a happy baby. This is why I've started the recipes as soon as the baby is born because a well-balanced, healthy diet will improve your energy levels and general well-being at a period when sleep, time, and patience are in extremely short supply. So I've kept it short and sweet. These recipes are easy to prepare and easily adapted. They are rich in vitamins, proteins, nutrients, and all-round goodness to keep you functioning at your peak. I've also tried to introduce some interesting tastes and flavors which may have dropped off your radar screen. Parents will be interested to read that babies' taste preferences are influenced by what their mother eats during breastfeeding. A study in 2001 (Manella, Jagnow & Beauchamp) showed that the babies of mothers who drank carrot juice while breastfeeding consumed more carrot-flavored baby rice. The more varied a mother's diet, the more likely it is that the baby will take to different foods during weaning.

Sing while you're weaning

If you've hit the weaning stage, you'll notice that all the recipes suggested are single variants of fruit or vegetables. I do this for a couple of reasons: First because giving them adult combinations like beef and vegetable risotto or lamb stew (as some commercial companies do) may be great for you after a busy day, but for a baby who has had nothing but milk it's going to be a bit of a struggle. The second reason is because it's a good way to monitor if there are any allergies. I suggest introducing each variant earlier in the day, either mid-morning or at lunchtime for a couple of days, to get your child used to them and give you time to check for any reactions. Then you can move on to another fruit or vegetable.

Shaping recipes

Wherever possible, I've created the recipes as single servings so you can try a small amount on your child without having to make large batches, but all recipes can be increased in size proportionately depending on how many children you have, how hungry they are or whether you have a moment to do a job lot and some home freezing. The recipes are intended as a starting point—feel free to change the ingredients using inspirations from the stage you are at or from previous stages. Just because a food is in stage 2 doesn't mean your baby shouldn't enjoy it at stages 3, 4 and beyond. The stage 2s, like peach, plum, and vanilla (wonderful with vanilla ice cream) and squash and red lentil (add a dash of pepper, maybe a little salt, and then a swirl of sour cream for a delicious adult soup), could be in your diet forever more. Going the other way, however, is a definite no-no. A stage 2 meal must not be given to a stage 1 baby. I've also shown you ways to use less common fruit and vegetables. So if your baby takes to them, adapt later stage recipes to incorporate them. Most of the recipes can be made into adult versions with a slight adaptation (or just a bit of seasoning) so you won't have to spend hours in the kitchen cooking for your children and then again for yourself.

Commercial baby foods

In a perfect world every parent would cook every meal from fresh organic produce. It would also put my company Fresh Daisy out of business. The reality is, even the busiest parent has days when time runs away from them and cooking meals from scratch is impossible.

Commercially available baby food fills the gap for days like these. Up until recently jars and cans have dominated the market. These are convenient because they can sit in the cupboard for two to three years and be pulled out in times of crisis. The problem for a parent who does most of their own cooking is that their child won't be familiar with the taste of this kind of food. Imagine cooking a piece of broccoli to 250°F in a pressure cooker and you'll begin to understand why

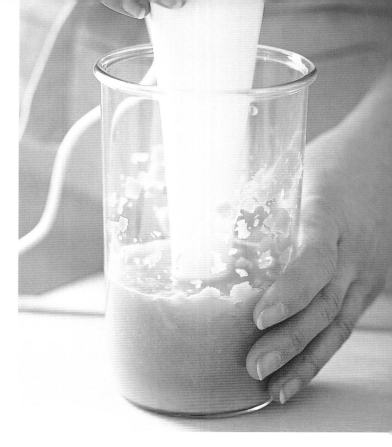

food from cans and jars loses its colour and texture and also tastes considerably different from homemade food.

Recently there has been a move toward yogurt-style pots. This is in reaction to the discovery of a potential cancer-causing carcinogen (semicarbazide) leaching from the jar's lid seal into the food. Despite the different format, the food is still sterilized and tastes the same as the jars and cans.

Frozen baby foods

For a product that replicates home cooking then frozen baby food (now being introduced in the USA), cooked from fresh (rather than concentrate), organic ingredients, is the best option. Freezing enables gentler cooking without destroying taste, color, and texture. You'll find it much easier to swap from good-quality frozen baby foods to homemade food since they will taste the same.

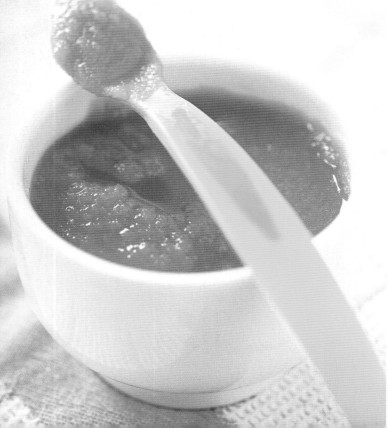

LEFT: **Carrot purée**, see page 60

Read the label

It's a good idea to get used to reading and understanding food labels to understand exactly what's going inside your baby's mouth. Since you've decided to buy *Naturally Delicious Meals for Baby* I guess you're keen to make as much homemade as possible—and that's the most obvious way to keep an eye on what goes into your and your baby's food, however, it's important to understand what is in the pre-packed alternatives. In the USA there are two governing bodies: The United States Food and Drug Administration (FDA) and the United States Department of Agriculture Food Safety Inspection Services (USDA FSIS) that are responsible for making sure domestic or imported foods are labelled with nutritional value and ingredients.

Nutritional Breakdown

Virtually all commercially available food has the nutritional breakdown listed. A few exceptions apply where food is prepared on-site, like in restaurants and fast food outlets, and for foods that have no nutritional value like coffee beans, tea, and food coloring. There are also around 300 staple products (like ketchup and peanut butter) which unless they deviate from standard ingredients are also exempt.

For the rest, the nutritional breakdown label usually includes the 14 nutrients including calories, calories from fat, saturated fats, cholesterol, sodium, total carbohydrate, dietary fiber, sugars, protein, and vitamins. Other nutrients are often voluntarily declared by the manufacturer.

However on baby food, especially in the first stages where there is only one or two ingredients, a simplified version is allowed containing core health information: calories, total fat sodium, carbohydrate, protein, vitamins, and minerals. You will also have noticed there is a Daily Value expressed as a percentage e.g in a $3^1/2$oz jar of carrot baby food you'd expect to see the following break-down: Protein: 2% Vitamin A: 55% Vitamin C: 0% Calcium: 4% Iron: 2%. It is a common misconception that

a low-fat, low-cholesterol, high-fiber diet is the perfect diet for children. It is right for adults but not for children under 4 years for fat is, in fact, very important for the healthy development of your baby—breast milk (or formula) and, after 12 months, dairy remain very important through the rapid-growth, developmental first four years of your child's life.

Additives

Major food manufacturers also like to jazz up foods to make them more attractive to consumers by using additives to give consumer-friendly colors and adding sweetness and flavoring to stop the product from going bad too quickly. Commercial baby food is very strictly regulated but for older children manufacturers will add sugar under different names so keep an eye out for sucrose, maltose, dextrose, fructose, maltodextrose, glucose, lactose, cane sugar, mannotose, corn syrup, inverted sugar, sugar syrup, and the rather cunningly named hydrolyzed starch.

Then there are the artificial sweeteners including aspartamine, acesulame K, and sucralose. These are all banned in foods specifically aimed at children under the age of 3 years so you won't find them lurking in a jar of baby food, but they are still present in all sorts of unlikely treats, snacks, ready meals, and soft drinks. An active child's diet does not have to be sugar free; they need the calories for energy—but as you will find in this book, there are ways to add natural sweetness to foods without lacing them with refined white sugar, syrups, or artificial sweeteners. If you're in any doubt, contact the FDA at www.fda.gov.

Why buy organic?

After months of feeding your little one a liquid lunch (and dinner, and breakfast ,and bed time snack!), watching them taste their first mouthful of solid food is as monumental a moment as their first word or step. Just as walking and talking require special nurturing and support, making sure your child develops a positive relationship with food is a fundamental responsibility of being a parent. You might assume feeding and watering your young one can't be too difficult (most people do it, don't they?), but with childhood obesity on the rise, increasing concerns about allergies and the mounting evidence linking poor diet with bad behavior, it's time to make some important decisions.

You might encounter a bit of a minefield of contradictory information while choosing the right food for your baby. The first major choice is the one between organic or non-organic. You're probably familiar with the organic sections of your supermarket and in the increasing number of health-food stores. You've probably also noticed that organic produce is more expensive, goes bad quicker, and the color and shape often don't compare to nonorganic. So why bother?

What price health?

The price we pay for slightly cheaper nonorganic vegetables is chemicals. There are almost 3,000 of them in our food chain. Conventional farming regularly uses a cocktail of chemicals to kill weeds, insects, and other pests to meet the tough cosmetic standards and a uniformity of size dictated by the chain stores. Take the common Delicious apple. You might think this is the perfect dessert, gently cooked, for your newly weaned baby, but just one apple could be sprayed up to 16 times with 36 different pesticides.

That's a problem because babies are even more susceptible to chemical residues than the average adult simply because they have a much higher intake of food and water per unit of body weight. Also, their tiny, immature digestive and immune systems mean they have a very limited ability to detoxify any chemical substances. Organic foods are free from pesticide contamination because synthetic chemicals are banned in organic farming, so I recommend using organic fruit and vegetables especially for children under 1 year of age—when they are at their most vulnerable. Although regulations for baby food manufacturers are extremely strict when it comes to micro-biological and chemical testing, I take the view that if the produce is organic it won't have chemicals at all instead of relying on chemical testing for known chemicals. Consider the Olympics and how athletes can get around the rules, and you'll see why I believe chemical testing is a safeguard but not an absolute. For me it's just not worth the risk.

Lifestyle choice

Beyond the food safety issue, there is the added bonus of supporting a way of farming that is not damaging the environment. Organic farming produces foods in fields that have been free from contaminants for a minimum of 3 years, rather than doctored with a cocktail of chemicals. And if all this is making you feel pretty good about yourself you'll be happy with the end-result in your shopping basket since organic food usually has a far superior taste, texture, and flavor to its non-organic rival.

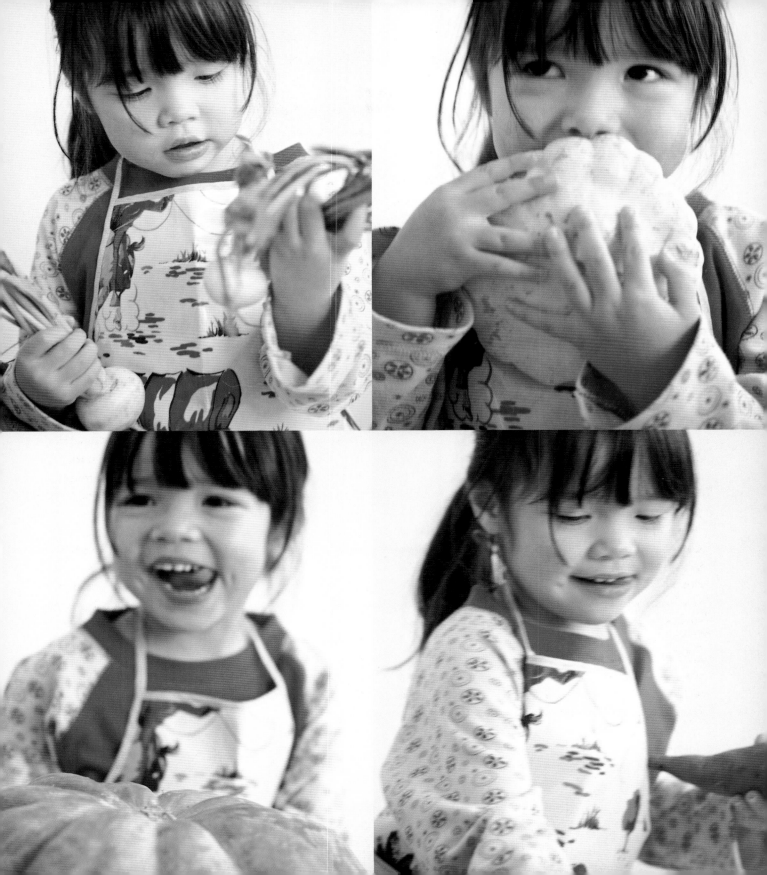

Quick-reference nutrition guide

Get yourself a cup of coffee, because, as they say in the shampoo commercials, this is the science part. Certain foods are important for your child's development and will help you to give your baby a balanced but varied diet. You may be able to reach for a chocolate bar or a package of potato chips when you're feeling hunger pangs, but unfortunately going dietary off-piste with your baby will lead to a seriously bumpy downhill run. So pay attention!

I've given a few examples of good food sources for each nutrient to help illustrate, though not all foods are suitable for a young baby. See page 21 and also each chapter for when to introduce what to your baby.

Carbohydrates

Or carbs, as they are now affectionately called in the post-Atkins era. We derive our energy and warmth from carbohydrates. When eaten they are broken down into glucose, which is carried to the muscles, brain, and other organs to enable us to function. Children need about five portions of carbohydrates a day and these should form about two-thirds of their diet.

Watch out, though, because there are bad carbs (simple carbs) and good carbs (complex carbs). Just imagine the story of the hare and the tortoise.

The hare and the tortoise

Simple carbs (the hare) include sugar, are most commonly found in refined foods (think cakes, white bread, cookies). They give a short, intense energy burst that disappears just as rapidly, leaving you craving more.

Complex carbs (the tortoise) include unrefined flours, grains, pulses, fruit, and vegetables. Because they are slower to digest than simple carbs, they release energy over a longer, more sustained period.

If your child eats too many simple carbs, their energy levels will yo-yo throughout the day. The refining process used to manufacture many of these carbs also strips foods of their vitamins and minerals. Take, for example, zinc, found in the outer layer of grain; if it's refined, the outer layer is stripped taking with it this valuable nutrient.

Food sources

Simple carbs cakes, white bread, white pasta, candy, white rice (see also section on sugar below).

Complex carbs vegetables, fruit, grains, pulses including lentils, whole-wheat flour, oats, rye or wholewheat bread, brown pasta, brown and wild rice (see also section on fiber on pages 17–18).

Fats

Fat has gotten some bad press. We all know we shouldn't eat too much, but we (and children especially) need to have fat of the right type and in the right amounts in our diets. Our bodies without fat are similar to a car grinding to a halt without oil; we need a small amount of certain fats to provide the essential lubricants that make us run smoothly inside and out.

Fats also go hand in hand with vitamins A, D, E, and K and minerals such as calcium.

Like carbs, there is "good" fat and "bad" fat:

Monounsaturated and polyunsaturated fats The good cops. As a rule of thumb you can recognize these as liquid at room temperature. Typically they are derived from fish, nuts, seeds, fruit, and vegetables. These essential fats are made up of essential fatty acids and are called essential because they are essential for life but can't be made by our own bodies.

Omega fatty acids

I'll give a special mention to the omega fatty acids: omega-3, omega-6 and their less well-known cousin omega-9. All are essential to life, but 3 and 6 can only be derived by eating foods containing them. Omega-9 can be produced by our bodies, though an additional supply from our diet is considered advisable. They all play an important role in our bodies whether we are children or adults, being necessary for supple skin, the development of the brain, growth of the nervous system and of muscle, protection from cancers... the list goes on.

For children, omega-3 is very important for brain development, improving the ability to concentrate. A recent study among elementary-school children in the U.K. who were given omega-3 supplements in their diets saw a remarkable change in school performance, with concentration levels improving by 35 percent.

Our diets tend to provide a plentiful supply of omega-6 oils but lack omega-3. The ideal ratio of omega-6 to omega-3 fats is 5:1, but ratios of omega-6 to omega-3 can be as imbalanced as 50:1.

Saturated fats The bad cops. As a quick rule of thumb they are recognizable as being solid at room temperature and typically come from animals (in meat or dairy)—though coconut and palm oil are also high in saturated fats.

Some saturated fat is good for children, especially as a warming extra energy source for the winter months. Too much will solidify in the body, clog up arteries, and form hard-to-shift stores in clumps around the body. Great. Although they provide an energy source, what makes them particularly nasty is the way they compete with the good cops, reducing the absorption of the essential oils.

Food sources

Monounsaturated and polyunsaturated fats oils from olives, avocados, fish, seeds (for older children, nuts).
omega-3 fatty acids are most readily found in fish, particularly oily fish (e.g. salmon, trout, mackerel, sardines, tuna). Some organic hens are now being fed a diet high in omega-3—providing organic free range eggs and chickens richer in omega-3 than average—particularly handy if your child dislikes oily fish. If you are choosing a vegetarian diet for your baby, you need to be particularly mindful of alternative omega-3 sources: tofu, linseed oil (flaxseed), ground linseed and for an older child, sunflower seeds, pumpkin seeds, sesame seeds and walnuts. See also Vegetarian babies on page 82.
omega-6 fatty acids almonds, pine nuts, avocados, corn, sunflower seeds, soya.
omega-9 fatty acids olive oils, avocados, some nut oils.
Saturated fats include red meat, butter, dairy products, and cheeses. They provide a good source of energy, but compete for absorption with the essential oils.

Proteins

Without proteins, we would be jelly. Proteins help to develop our skeletons and muscles as we grow and maintain our body tissues. They also act as messengers between the brain, nervous and hormonal systems. Initially children need more protein per pound of body weight than a fully grown adult. Proteins are broken down into amino acids in the digestive tract then dispersed around the body to help build and rebuild every cell in our body. Proteins are made up of 22 amino acids, 8 of which are "essential" (we don't make them ourselves, so we need to eat them). Meat, fish, and dairy contain the full spectrum of amino acids we need; however it is harder work to get the full amino acid set if you're a vegetarian.

Food sources

Meat, poultry, fish, dairy as well as eggs, seeds, grains especially quinoa, beans, and pulses including lentils, soy, and soy-based foods such as tofu. Nuts are also protein rich but can be allergenic: see Avoiding allergies, pages 56–7.

Fiber

Fiber, along with the right amount of fluid, keeps food on the move through your bowels. Most adults could do with increasing the amount of fiber they eat, while older children also need a fiber-rich diet instead of one based on refined foods because without it our systems become sluggish and constipated. However, roughage can be too coarse for a baby's bowels and that's why early weaning foods are peeled and cooked: it's the peel rather than the flesh of fruit and vegetables that contains the most roughage.

There are two types of fiber, both of which are needed to keep things moving:

Insoluble fiber (also called roughage) helps to sweep the colon and is important in adults and older children. Young bowels can find these abrasive.

Soluble fiber maintains some bulk in the bowels: see Poop, page 29.

Food sources
Insoluble fiber wheat and other grain husks, oats, skin of fruit and vegetables, unrefined (brown) flour, rice, pasta.
Soluble fiber fruits, vegetables, beans, and pulses.

Sugars
Sugar is a simple carbohydrate and is a huge issue in children's diets as one of the worst culprits in the obesity epidemic. Why? When your blood sugar goes up, you produce more insulin. And the more insulin you produce, the more sugar you keep as fat. Sugar is very, very addictive and can send moods and energy levels on a rollercoaster ride—the lows causing us to crave more and so the cycle continues. But hold on, sugar is composed of a group of simple carbohydrates and the problem is mainly caused by the kind of sugar that is spooned into and on to food. Soft drinks can contain about 8 teaspoons of refined sugar and most jelly-like candies are virtually pure sugar—it's highly refined from sugar cane and sugar beets, of little nutritional value and one of the main causes of tooth decay.

Fruit and, to a lesser extent, milk, and vegetables contain natural sugars and should provide enough sweetness for adults and children alike. In a child's first year you should not add any extra sugar to their food—just use the natural sweetness of the pure ingredients.

Keep an eye out for added sugars when you're doing your supermarket shopping since they are found in many processed foods. Sugars are known by other aliases, including glucose syrup, sucrose, maltose, fructose, and dextrose. For more on sugars, see Read the label on page 13.

Honey is seen as a natural alternative to sugar but is a big no-no for babies under 12 months. Never use it to sweeten baby food—this is not because of nutrition but for food safety reasons. In rare cases, honey can contain spores of the bacteria *Clostridium botulinum*, which can cause serious food poisoning or infant botulinum, a very nasty bacteria infection that infants are susceptible to. You may find that some commercial baby food manufacturers use honey to sweeten recipes unnecessarily—they can do this because the extreme temperatures needed to process the food destroys the bacteria but consequently damages the purées' taste, texture, and color.

Salt
Salt is the common name for sodium chloride and is also being eyed by food experts as a serious player in the rising obesity problem. It may be that high levels of salt make certain foods so attractive, triggering a reaction in our bodies that makes us crave them. It's notable most junk foods, ready meals, and many of our favorite snacks are laden with flavour-enhancing salt.

Salt should never be added to food for a baby under 12 months old because their kidneys are not able to cope with it. All baby food manufacturers are required to adhere to this advice when formulating their products.

As adults, the amount of salt we like in our food can creep up without us really noticing, so as you start to make and taste baby food you may initially find it bland. Accept that it's salt free, and you might be surprised at how you also start to reexperience the real taste of the pure foods you are preparing. The addition of herbs and spices is a flavoursome alternative to adding salt.

Salt is rarely listed on the labels of foods; instead it will be included under the heading sodium. Sodium occurs naturally in a wide variety of foods and some sodium is essential in the diet, but a normal, mixed diet will provide your infant with all the sodium they require without the need for any added salt.

Vitamins and minerals

Vitamins and minerals are essential for well-being and work quietly behind the scenes to make sure everything is A-O.K. Vitamins are either water soluble (they dissolve in water), like vitamin B and C, or fat soluble (they are stored in the liver and fat tissues of your body), like vitamins A, D, E, and K. Water-soluble vitamins travel through your body, coming out in urine, and need to be guzzled daily, while fat-soluble vitamins are stored by the body for up to six months and called on as needed.

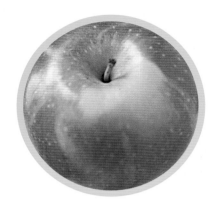

Vitamin A (beta-carotene)
What does it do?
Builds good eyesight (helps you to see in the dark), keeps skin soft and smooth, a must for your immune system, needed for gleaming teeth, hair, and nails and important for maintaining the health of the thyroid gland.
Food sources Orange/red fruit and vegetables, e.g. carrots, red peppers, sweet potatoes, pumpkin and squash, peaches, tomatoes, egg yolk, oily fish, whole milk.

Vitamin B (thiamin, riboflavin, niacin, pantothenic acid, pyridoxine, cyanocobalamin, folic acid)
What does it do?
Vitamin B is actually a group of vitamins (B^1, B^2, B^3, B^5, B^6, B^{12}, folic acid, and biotin). In general terms they help to convert food into energy, keep our stomachs and intestines healthy, and help to prevent infections. Specifically, B^1 and B^2 help to break down food and stave off infection; B^3 builds brain cells; B^5 helps to maintain red blood cells; B^6 helps to produce antibodies to fight disease; B^{12} is essential for the development of the central nervous system. Folic acid is essential for blood formation, and in pregnancy it helps to prevent neural tube defects, such as spina bifida; also essential for the development of the central nervous system.
Food sources A balanced diet! Whole grains, pulses, green leafy vegetables, dairy, eggs, oily fish, red meat; for older kids: nuts, brewers' yeast, and yeast extract—note this is high in salt, so not recommended for those under 12 months.

Vitamin C (ascorbic acid)
What does it do?
Vitamin C helps to fight infection and to absorb iron. It's important for healing, acts as an antioxidant (offers protection against free-radical damage that can precipitate cancer, heart disease, and other conditions). It is essential for building muscles and cartilage.
Food sources All fruit (particularly berries, kiwi fruit, citrus fruits, strawberries). All red, green, and yellow vegetables (particularly red and yellow sweet peppers, tomatoes, and broccoli).

Vitamin D (calciferol)
What does it do?
Helps the absorption of calcium and phosphorus as well as helping to strengthen bones and teeth.
Food sources With the increase in the incidence of skin cancer, many of us are keeping out of the sun; however, a little sun is essential for making vitamin D. If sun is a no go, try oily fish, liver, egg yolk, and butter.

Vitamin E
What does it do?
Contains anti-aging properties, necessary for healthy cell membranes. Also helps to protect certain fatty acids.
Food sources Wheatgerm, avocado, nuts, seeds.

Vitamin K

What does it do?

Helps the blood to clot (which is needed for wounds to heal); essential to build strong bones and prevent heart disease.

Food sources Green leafy vegetables; also manufactured by the body from gut bacteria.

Calcium

What does it do?

Essential for bones and teeth. Breastfeeding women need it in abundance, but keep in mind that it needs vitamin D to be absorbed.

Food sources All dairy foods (particularly hard cheese and milk), lentils, whole small fish, sunflower seeds, green vegetables, mangoes.

Iron

What does it do?

Essential for the formation of red blood cells; low levels of iron result in anemia (symptoms include tiredness, lethargy, low energy levels, breathlessness, tingling hands). Iron absorption can be increased by 30 percent if combined with vitamin C-rich foods, but calcium reduces the uptake of iron.

Food sources Kidneys, liver, meats, shellfish, egg yolks, dried apricots, prunes, pumpkin seeds, haricot beans, raisins.

Zinc

What does it do?

Helps the formation of many enzymes and proteins as well as moving vitamin A from liver stores into the bloodstream.

Food sources Red meat, eggs, liver, nuts, onions, shellfish, sunflower seeds, wheat germ, whole wheat.

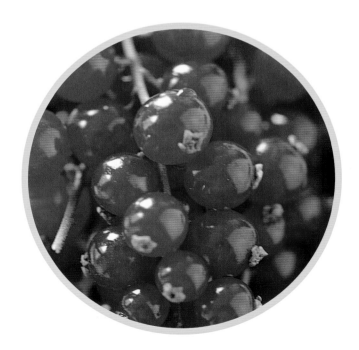

When to introduce certain foods into your baby's diet

Stage 1 should not be started before 4 months (see note below), stage 2 should not be started before 6 months, stage 3 is for 9 months and onward, and stage 4 for 12 months and onward.

	Preweaning	Stage 1	Stage 2	Stage 3	Stage 4
Vegetables	No	Peeled, cooked, and puréed until smooth—see stage 1 recipes.	Peeled, cooked, and puréed with texture—see stage 2 recipes.	Cooked and raw finger foods.	
Fruit	No	Peeled, cooked, and puréed until smooth—see stage 1 recipes.	Peeled, cooked, and puréed with some texture—see stage 2 recipes. Some raw purées.	Cooked and raw finger foods.	
Milk and Dairy	Breast or formula milk will remain important throughout the first year.		Add toward end of stage: cooked milk, yogurts, hard-boiled eggs, hard cheese.		After 12 months, whole pasteurized milk to drink.
Fish	No	No	Introduce toward the end of this stage. Not smoked.		
Smoked Fish	No	No	No	No	In moderation.
Shellfish	No	No	No	No	Only if well cooked.
Gluten	No	No	No	In moderation.	
Meat and Chicken	No	No	Toward the end of this stage (avoiding high salt e.g. bacon, ham).		
Berries	No	No	Can be introduced if mashed or puréed. Monitor for any reactions.		
Sugar and Artificial Sweeteners	No	No	No	No	If foods need to be sweetened, use fruit purées from stage 1.
Fiber (High)	No	No	No	No	As part of a balanced diet.
Salt	No	No	No	No	Food contains salt, so no need to add extra.
Tofu	No	No	Toward the end of this stage.		
Nuts	No	No	No	No	Avoid whole nuts (choking hazard). Introduce ground or as a paste. Monitor for any reactions.
Citrus	No	No	No	Can be introduced.	
Honey	No	No	No	No	After 12 months.

- Exclusive breastfeeding is recommended for the first 6 months. If you want to start weaning earlier than 6 months you should consult your pediatrician. Weaning earlier than 4 months is known to be detrimental to the health of a baby.
- If your family has a history of allergies to certain foods, you should avoid introducing them until you have consulted your pediatrician.

Cooking and storing

Once you get started, you'll soon discover that there is a basic pattern to the recipes, especially in the early stages. This is an overview of the method and a quick explanation about why you're doing what.

Wash Fruit and vegetables (especially root vegetables) need a good clean if you're using nonorganic produce since they are the most susceptible to contamination from chemicals and pesticides. Because organic produce is not allowed to be sprayed, you may find the odd bug, especially in broccoli and cauliflower.

Peel This is important because too much roughage can be too harsh on babies' developing internal systems. Skins are also the most exposed to contamination by handling, so peeling is a good safeguard in the first two stages.

Chop The secret to a tasty end result, especially in the early stage purées, is in the size of the pieces. If they vary or are too big, they will end up overcooked. I recommend a ¼ inch dice for most fruit and vegetables. Use immediately after chopping because the nutrients start to deteriorate.

Cook Steaming retains the natural flavors and textures of the ingredients. Adding food to boiling water, rather than cooking from cold, also staves off nutrient deterioration. Certain meals and fruits and vegetables lend themselves to pan cooking, but you can adapt most of the recipes to the cooking utensils you have in your kitchen.

Blend This enables you to control the textures you give to your baby, which is extremely important in the first two weaning stages. Watch out for potatoes: They need only a quick blend or the starches come out and make purées gluey, which is why some parents prefer to serve as a mash.

Sieve In the early stages, pushing the purée through a sieve using the back of a spoon, or using a fine food mill disk will give you a very smooth end-product. Once through this initial stage, you can use a coarser disk, which will give you a thicker texture, without the worry of any choking hazards sneaking through. Watch out for bananas because they'll end up as a gray sludge if you try to sieve them.

Cool Always allow the food to cool, and then test it yourself to make sure it is the right temperature to serve to your baby. If you want to store some of the food in the fridge or freezer, cover and cool first as heat can reduce the efficiency of your fridge or freezer. Don't leave food out at room temperature, especially rice, meats, and fish, since this is the most dangerous procedure for producing bacteria (see page 27 for details on freezing).

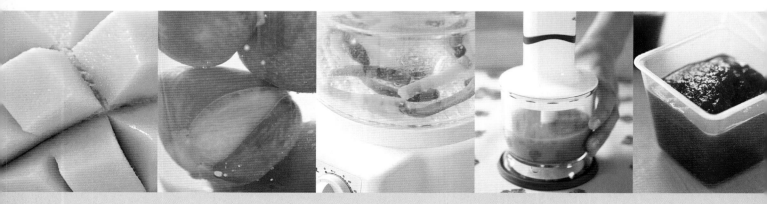

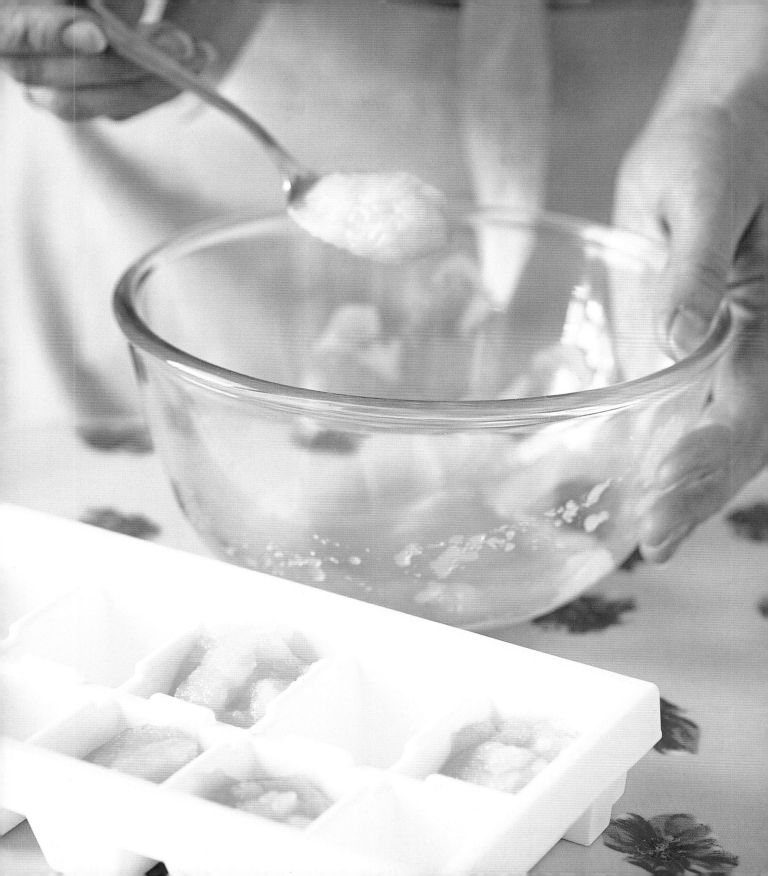

Equipment

There are now a huge array of products available for kitting out your baby. There are parents whose priority is to dress their mini-me head to toe in Gucci (good for them), but parents should also appreciate that food is crucial at all stages of development, so getting the right equipment to encourage your child along is imperative. You may already have some of this equipment in your kitchen, but here are a few pointers to help you choose what to buy.

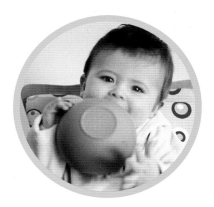

For babies
Weaning spoons Metal conducts heat, so always choose a plastic spoon, preferably one with a long handle and a shallow bowl with blunt sides.

Weaning bowls Look out for small, plastic bowls. Try a bowl with two compartments so you can put carrot purée in one side and apple in the other and mix the two together as the meal goes on. Or try one food you know they eat and introduce a new one.

Bibs Draping a clean dish towel is equally effective as a cotton bib. For trainee spoon users, a plastic bib with a trough will help to catch bits. Bibs with a plastic backing will protect clothes from getting wet or stained.

Bouncy chair or Bumbo In the first stages of weaning before your baby is ready for a high chair, use a bouncy chair or a plastic Bumbo seat to support their back. It will also keep your hands free.

High chair If your baby has full head control and a strong back, it's time for a high chair. High chairs that can be pulled right up to the table and be adjusted as your child grows are the best. Chairs like this make them feel part of the whole mealtime party. They love it. Make sure they are safely fastened in so they can't wriggle and fall out. Some babies get fed up with being in the chairs for too long, so don't hoist them up until the meal is ready.

For toddlers
Toddler-friendly cutlery Choose varieties with a short handle that is easy to hold (some come with grips). Novelty train and airplane spoons are a cunning idea and will help to distract fussy feeders.

Toddler plates You can buy ones that come with individual compartments, which can appeal to picky eaters as well as create a come-hither-looking meal, or you can just use toddler-friendly nondivided plates. Some plates come with a funny picture—an incentive for your child to get to the bottom of the food.

For the kitchen
Ice cube trays and tiny-freezer containers These are a must. When you've made your purée, simply portion it into the pots or trays and use as needed. Cover ice cube trays with a freezer bag before freezing. You can reuse some store containers and some yogurt pots (sterilize them first, see page 26). When using plastic cups or ice cube trays, make sure they are sealed tight as they can be contaminated by other products in the freezer.

Small freezer bags and a marker pen Decant the frozen cubes into small, single-serving bags and mark with the purée variety and date, so you can easily identify them later.

Hand-held electric blender These are a godsend; seek out an electric blender pack which includes a small chopping bowl and blade: These are fantastic for tiny stage 1 quantities and getting a very smooth texture. As your child gets older, you can simply purée cooked vegetables in the saucepan (and economize on dishes).

Food processor Although these are rarely able to create very fine purées for fledging foodies, food processors are handy for stage 2 purées. They come into their own for fine-chopping large quantities quickly.

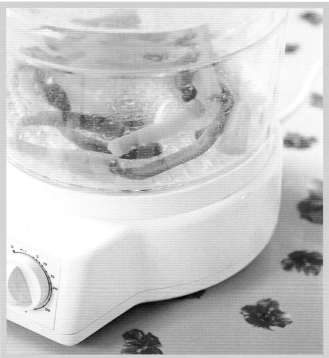

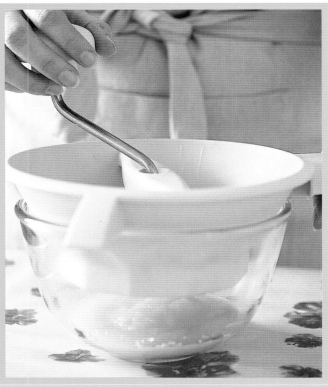

Food mill This is a food mill you can turn by hand (see photograph left), is particularly good for giving stage 1 purées a reassuring final sieve. It's ideal for tough-skinned foods, such as prunes, dried apricots, peas, and fava beans, since it produces an even purée by keeping out coarse fibrous parts (like husks or skins).

Electric steamer An electric steamer with timer switch and stock-collecting tray (see photograph above) will save you time, deliver the best flavor, and, unlike a saucepan, they don't have to be watched in case they boil over. I'm a big fan.

Chopping boards Raw meat and fish should have a separate board from cooked. Rather than clutter up your kitchen, check out small, dishwasher-friendly chopping boards, in different colors to help you to remember which one is for what.

Hygiene and sterilization

Food hygiene for babies

When it comes to preparing food for babies, cleanliness is next to godliness. If you've been a slob in your prebaby existence, now is the time to shape up—you might be able to withstand the bacteria of week-long leftovers, but your baby will not. Their immune system is only just developing and needs you to take extra care and attention in the kitchen. A bout of food poisoning could make them very ill indeed. So get out the mop, throw away those yucky old dishcloths, and review a few golden rules.

The fridge

Make sure the fridge temperature is set between 32 and 41°F and the freezer should be no warmer than 4°F. (Fridge and freezer thermometers are available from most department stores.)

Store your baby's food (and bottles) in the middle of the fridge. Avoid the door compartment (the warmest part of the fridge) and the very back since it can be cold enough to freeze.

Always put raw meat at the bottom of the fridge, so that the juices can't drip down and contaminate other food in the fridge.

Sterilizing and cleaning

Now that every stray toy, book, or shoe is heading straight for your baby's mouth, there's not much point in sterilizing anything other than their eating and drinking utensils (console yourself with the knowledge that babies need a few germs to build up their defenses). What you can do is:

Wash all baby's plates and utensils in the dishwasher on the hottest cycle or invest in a pair of rubber gloves and wash in very hot water, then rinse in clean water, ideally over 140°F, and air dry.

Regularly mop the floors and wipe down the high chair before and after every meal.

Clean all surfaces using a nontoxic sterilizing fluid diluted according to the manufacturer's instructions—there are several brands available already diluted in handy spray bottles for added convenience and speed.

Don't skimp on dishcloths—dirty damp cloths can spread bacteria through the kitchen. Wash them regularly on the hottest machine setting or use disposable cloths and throw them away.

Change your dish-towels every day or more often if dirty.

Preparing food

By following a few guidelines, you'll know that your baby (or your kitchen floor, at least) is getting both the freshest and healthiest food there is.

Wash your hands with soap before starting (15 seconds under warm, running water is a good guideline).

Use separate boards for cutting meat and vegetables—ideally rigid plastic ones. Don't use wooden ones because they are porous and retain bacteria. Scrub them down in hot water after use and allow to air dry.

Wash fruit and vegetables thoroughly and peel if they are not organic; this will protect your baby against pesticides.

Freezing, defrosting, and reheating

If you are freezing baby food, small bags are best since they are sealable. If you are using ice cube trays be extremely careful because leaving them uncovered in the freezer leaves them open to contamination from the other products being stored. Check out the great individual cube molds with lids (see photograph right).

Always label and date food so you know what it is and when it needs to be thrown away (fruit, vegetable, and meat purées can be kept for up to 3 months; fish, grains and pulses for 2).

Reheat food until it is piping hot, then allow to cool before serving to your baby. Always be very careful with rice. If left for several hours at room temperature, cooked rice can cause food poisoning. Further cooking or reheating will not destroy the bacteria. Either keep rice hot (at or above 145°F), or refrigerated, or frozen. If using baby rice always make small amounts fresh each time as you require.

Do not reheat foods more than once and never refreeze uneaten food.

ABOVE RIGHT: **Beet purée,** see page 66

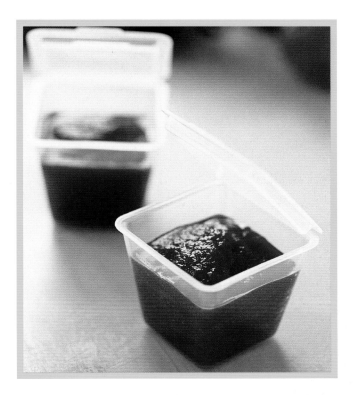

Finger foods

Life will get easier as your baby starts to eat more of what you do, but there are still a few rules to remember:

Never leave food in open cans. Transfer leftovers into a closeable container, store in the refrigerator, and eat within 48 hours.

Babies are particularly susceptible to salmonella, so cook eggs until the white and yolk are solid.

Don't offer a medium-rare option—cook all meat until the juices run clear.

Look at the use-by date on all products.

And finally, if you're concerned about any food for any reason, DON'T GIVE IT TO YOUR BABY!

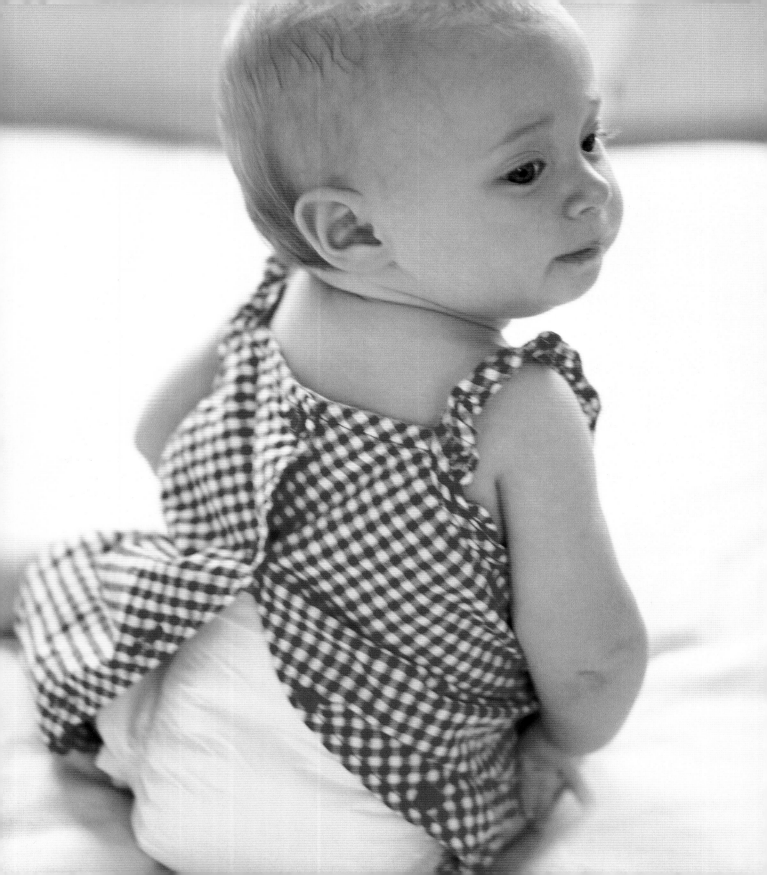

Poop

OK, stop snickering, we all do it (yes, even the president) and when it comes to your child (and even you), it's a great way of checking to see if everything is working properly. Think of your baby as a little production unit. If food passes through their system too quickly (diarrhea) or slowly (constipation), then the unit is not going to operate properly and your baby is not getting the best out of their food. So have your clipboard ready and put your supervisor's hat on because here's a quick guide to poop. Bet they didn't teach you about this in school!

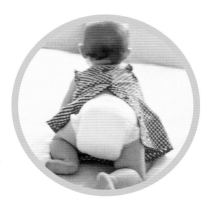

As you start to wean your baby, you'll soon notice that their poop will change drastically in color and smell from the mustard-color of milk-only poop to the more "human-looking" logs.

When first weaning, your baby may find some foods hard to digest. And because you're feeding one vegetable at a time (for example beets), you may find their poop will be colored like the food (a beet eater's poop can be very red). Don't be alarmed—it's perfectly natural (but a bit of a nightmare for the diapers!).

Your baby may find it hard to pass some of their first foods. Baby rice, for example, can clog up little bowels, as can bananas. If your baby is really straining (going red in the face, eyes bulging, even crying) you may need to alter their diet and liquid intake.

Helping things along

Ways to prevent poop from being too dry and hard is to give your baby more fruit (particularly pears) or boiled water (in a beaker or bottle) when feeding. Prune purée (see page 74), served alone, or mixed in with fruit or baby rice, or diluted prune juice is another way of gently getting those bowels to work. Hard poop may be a sign that your baby is not getting enough to drink: add a little formula, or breast milk, or cooking water to loosen their food—and bowels—up. To help the elimination process, make sure your baby gets some exercise each day since being stuck in a baby carriage for too long can also jam them up. When "exercising" take their diaper off and let them kick around under a baby gym or on a big mat with toys just out of reach, or put them on their tummy for a while.

Speeding things up or slowing them down

If your toddler is constipated, it may be that they need to eat a little more fiber, so swap white bread for brown, white pasta for whole-wheat, and include fiber-filled beans or lentils until the problem has resolved itself. If all else fails, a burst of exercise and fresh air (travel, change, illness, and stress are clogging culprits) may do the trick.

Diarrhea is another issue, but the causes can be quite varied. It can be related to an illness, a food sensitivity, or an indication that your baby is eating too much fruit or fiber. Tiny tots can get dehydrated very quickly so make sure they keep up their fluid intake with diluted noncitrus fruit juice. If the diarrhea is really bad, you may need oral rehydrating salts available from your drugstore; ask your pharmacist or doctor for advice. After a bout of diarrhea, give your little one food that is easy to digest and kind to the gut; for example rice, banana, toast, pear purée, sweet potatoes, and live natural yogurt (this helps to rebuild lost gut flora).

Tastes from day one

A healthy, protein-packed diet will help you cope during this energy-sapping stage and give breastfeeding babies a taste of things to come.

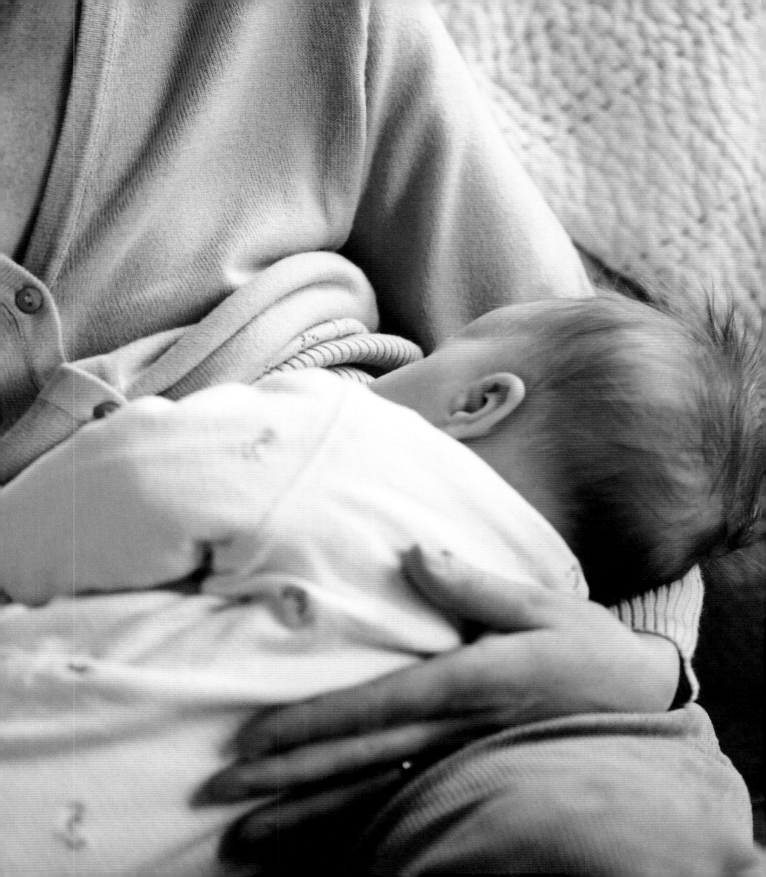

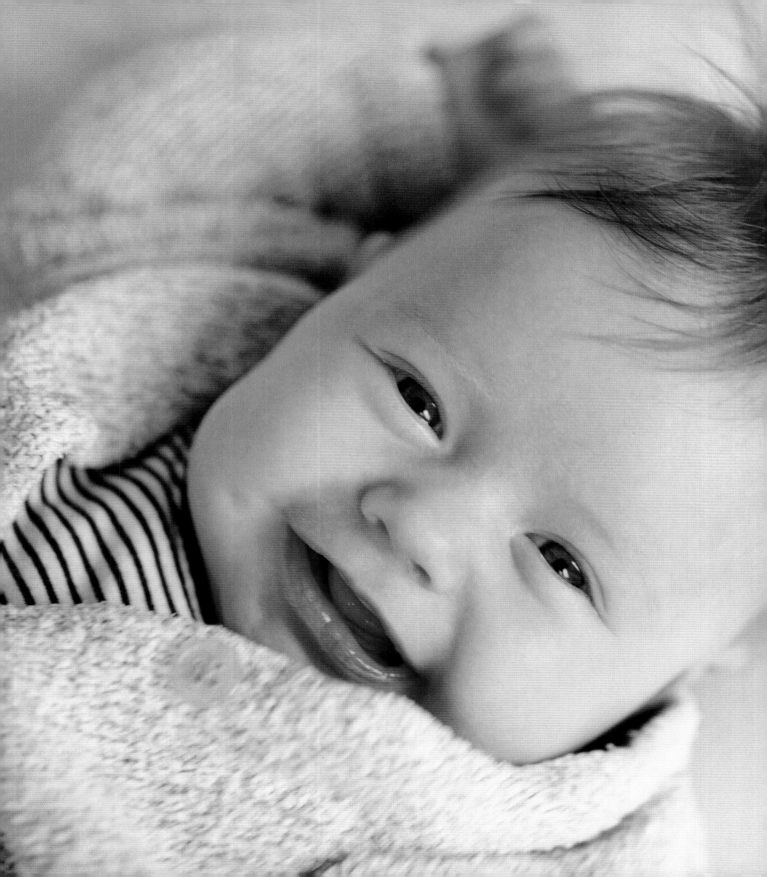

Milk, milk, glorious milk

There's no escaping from it and here it comes again in big bold letters: Breast is best. Breast milk provides your baby with all their nutritional needs. Yes, your milk is perfectly concocted for your baby. The benefits of breastfeeding are endless. From the creamy first milk of colostrum— high in protein, vitamins, minerals, and antibodies—to your everyday breast milk, your own milk changes with your baby's needs. And, what's more, as you vary what you eat, it comes in a variety of flavors (and even color tints) too.

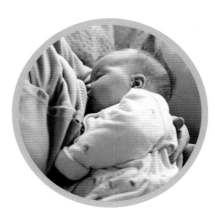

Breastfeeding

A varied, nutritious diet helps to create a good milk supply and also lays the foundation for your baby's tastebuds. The good news is you don't have to follow the perfect diet to produce great milk. Nature is fabulously forgiving. Women in famine conditions produce perfectly good breast milk, but eventually the body draws on its own reserves, which can result in deficiencies for the mother. In general, mineral levels (iron, copper, chromium, zinc) are stable in human milk regardless of maternal blood levels.

Eating for two

To maintain an abundant supply of milk, most women need around 1,800–2,200 calories a day. If you consume fewer, your milk supply could drop. On average, an exclusively breastfeeding mother needs to consume about 300–500 calories a day more than she used to before her pregnancy. Most women put on lovely maternal fat stores during pregnancy which contribute about 200 extra calories a day toward lactation, so it may be that you only need one or two extra snacks a day.

What food should you avoid? Although advice will say you can include all the things you've put a hold on while pregnant, overdoing the rich foods may make your baby colicky. If your own or your partner's family has an allergy history with a certain food, avoid them—if in any doubt, nuts and especially peanuts could also be worth avoiding (see pages 56–7).

If you are attempting breastfeeding but finding it harder than you expected, you're not alone. Talk to your doctor—there may be a fantastic breastfeeding counselors you can be referred to. For everything you need to know about breastfeeding, go to the National Women's Health Information: www.4women.gov/breastfeeding or breastfeeding experts at www.lalecheleague.org.

First tastes for your baby

Your newborn baby cries, whimpers, wails as they shout, "Fill me up, Mom," at every breakfast, lunch, dinner, and midnight snack. Milk is all your baby wants—and, in the early months, it's all your baby needs.

Yet these months are more than just a milky whitewash and your little gourmet is forming taste preferences before they even have a tooth. That means, and it's a big one, everything, yes everything you eat while breastfeeding is influencing your baby's taste preferences. Research has shown that a baby's tastebuds may even be shaped in the womb by the flavor of your amniotic fluid, which acts as a "flavor bridge" to breast milk.

Breast milk is also a "flavor bridge" to food and, depending on what you eat, your milk will come in an array of mouth-watering flavors. This isn't a new discovery. Medical documents from as far back as the fourteenth century state that a mother's milk could be more pleasant if the mother ate sweet foods or imbibed fragrant wines (presumably in moderation!). On the other hand, salty or seasoned meats and particular spices would cause her milk to become "heated" and "acrimonious."

In 2004, a research study at the Monell Institute in Philadelphia showed that breastfed babies with mothers who have a varied diet are much more likely to accept unfamiliar flavors when weaned and are more willing to try new vegetables than their formula-fed friends. Another study showed that when garlic flavors are present in breast milk, babies are inclined to suck for longer, but when alcohol is present, they suck more quickly initially, but drink less and finish faster. As you breastfeed you may find your baby relishes some flavors and rejects others. Watch what you eat, then see how long they suck for—keep an eye out for foods that could make your milk bitter as babies innately reject bitter tastes (it's a lifesaving reflex as many natural poisons are bitter to taste). A hit of strong coffee will flavor your milk within 30 minutes.

Why breast milk is great for your baby
- Breast milk is a nutritionally complete food for your baby.
- Human milk provides your baby's first set of living immune cells.
- Human milk has special ingredients, e.g. DHA (docosohexaenoic acid) and AA (arachidonic acid), which contribute to brain and eye development.
- Breast milk gives your baby the first tastes of real food.
- Mothers who breastfeed for 6 months have a reduced risk of breast cancer.
- Mothers who breastfeed lose their maternal fat stores faster than those who bottlefeed.

Bottlefeeding and formula milk
Before formula, the only alternative to breast milk was another mother's milk. A wet nurse was the only milk substitute. In the Middle Ages it was believed a wet nurse's vices could be sucked through their milk, so candidates were always carefully selected—hair coloring, for example, was then viewed with suspicion. Animal milk wasn't even considered until the eighteenth century, for if a child's temperament could come from a human's milk, just imagine what kind of characteristics they might inherit from a cow! In fact, normal cow's milk is too high in protein and salt to be used without modification for any infant under a year.

These days formula milk manufacturers give cow's milk a human-friendly makeover to make it suitable for babies under 1 year, by modifying the carbohydrates, proteins, and fats in animal milk and adding vitamins and minerals including folic acid, zinc, and iron.

Alternatives to dairy formula milk
The alternatives to milk formula include soybean-based formula, but this is not recommended for babies under 6 months. Lactose intolerance in babies is rare, but signs to watch out for include abdominal pain and swelling, gas, and diarrhea. If your baby is experiencing these symptoms seek medical advice for alternative formulas—these may only be available on prescription.

Choose organic
When selecting a formula, check the labels and choose organic formulas whenever you can. The formulas are made from cows that haven't been given growth hormones and are reared in organic meadows, so the milk is less likely to carry harmful chemical or pesticide residues. As always, keep everything pristine clean since milk is a fertile breeding ground for bacteria. When you use new bottles, rings, or nipples, always sterilize them first.

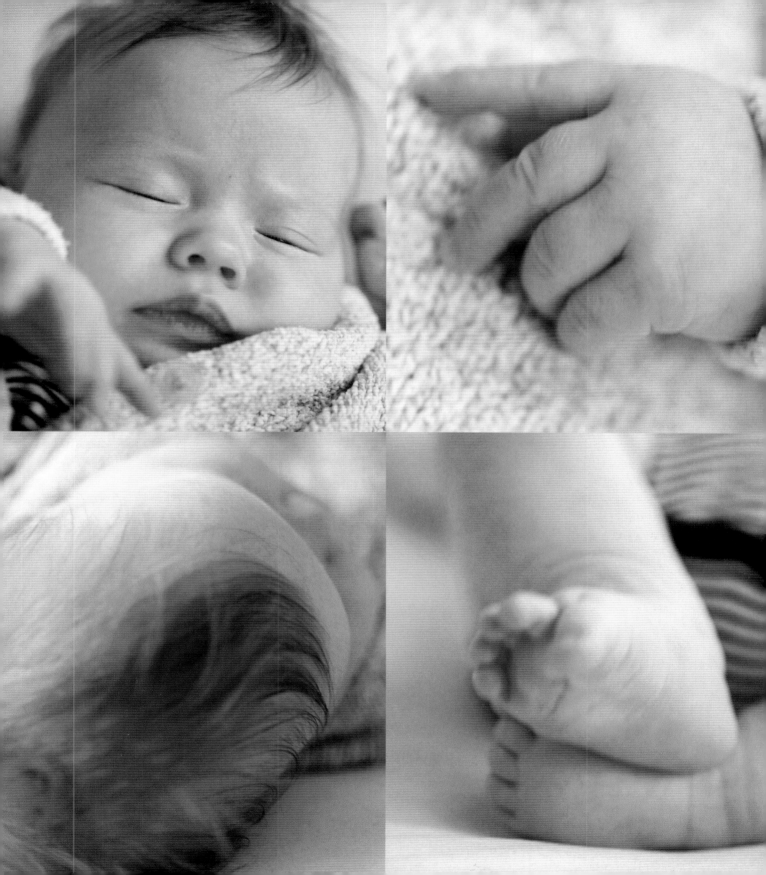

The big breakfast

Lunch may be for wimps but breakfast is a meal even Sylvester Stallone would struggle to do without. Skipping breakfast, then running on empty will result in a serious breakdown before lunchtime. And just so we know where we stand, three strong coffees, back to back, do not constitute a healthy breakfast! These days breakfast is more likely to be a quick fill-'er-up on the run, rather than a relaxed breakfast in bed with a magazine, but if you choose simple, easy-to-prepare meals you can eat all the energy-packed foods you need to get you through the day.

Having your breakfast on a silver tray is probably restricted to a time your partner is trying to get out of the doghouse, but one thing remains a constant and that's the importance of a good breakfast. Those who eat a proper breakfast work faster, make fewer mistakes, suffer fewer colds, and have a better short-term memory. What's more, they are less likely to have vitamin or mineral deficiencies.

Without breakfast, hunger levels soar and energy levels plummet by mid-morning, which is when we reach for high-energy foods or overindulge at lunchtime. Skipping breakfast means you are more likely to have a higher body mass index.

Food for the brain

Breakfast is also vital brain fodder. Researchers in Scotland found that consuming a breakfast rich in complex carbohydrates benefits short-term memory by supplying the brain with a steady supply of glucose. Children who eat a breakfast rich in complex carbs improved their memory performance throughout the morning. U.S. researchers found that children who don't eat breakfast have problems with basic problem-solving skills, verbal fluency, and the ability to recall facts.

What is a good breakfast?

What to eat? We all bow to Maximilian Bircher-Benner, the creator of "Birchermüsli" at his Living Force Clinic in 1900. His cereal, made originally from grated apple, lemon juice, milk, nuts, and grains, was "prescribed" as a protection against illness of all kinds (this is now backed up by a study from the University of Wales, which reveals that those who eat breakfast are less likely to suffer from colds and flu). Muesli is probably the only Swiss-German word to have gone global. It's a meal in one, loaded with vitamin C (fresh fruits), calcium (yogurt, milk), protein (nuts or seeds), iron (dried apricots and prunes), and more. Not only is it great with milk, you can also turn it into crumble topping or create nutritious snacks like granola bars or muffins for your toddlers.

Full Monty Muesli—Real Swiss Style

The original Birchermüsli, though wholesome, could also be described as a bit too worthy. These days if you ask for a Birchermüsli, you can expect a delicious fruity, yogurty, oaty bowl of loveliness that will fill you up and feel like a treat without the guilt trip of a full breakfast.

Makes 1 serving (not suitable for freezing)

THE NIGHT BEFORE
1 tablespoon rolled oats
3 tablespoons water

JUST BEFORE SERVING
1–2 tablespoons yogurt, cream, or crème fraîche
1 apple

1 tablespoon mixed berries and currants (fresh or, if out of season, frozen)
1 piece of seasonal fruit, e.g. peach, apricot, pear
1 tablespoon lemon juice
1 tablespoon chopped seeds or nuts (traditionally hazelnuts)

Soak the oats in the water overnight—it makes them easier to digest.

Shortly before serving, mix the oats with the yogurt, cream, or crème fraîche. Wash, core, and grate the unpeeled apple and chop the other fruits as necessary. Stir into the mix. If you like, toast the seeds and nuts (if you are not allergic) and sprinkle on to the mix.

Serve immediately.

Tropical Oatmeal

This is a tropical version, although the same method works with more locally available seasonal fruit. Two brazil nuts a day provide the recommended daily allowance of the mood-enhancing mineral selenium—though omit if you are adapting this recipe for a child.

Makes 1 serving (not suitable for freezing)

½ cup milk
a handful of rolled oats
1 tablespoon dried or fresh mango, papaya, and pineapple
1 tablespoon dried coconut

2 chopped brazil nuts
1 small banana

Pan method
Heat the milk in a small pan and stir in the oats, bring to a boil, and return to a simmer.

Stir in the fruit and nuts, if using, and cook for 10–12 minutes until the oats are soft. Pour into a bowl and top with banana—which will help to cool it slightly.

Microwave method (and dish-washing-saving method)
Combine all the ingredients except the banana in a large, microwave-safe, breakfast bowl. (Choose a bowl bigger than you think needed since it tends to bubble up and can boil over.)

Cook for 1 minute on full power, stir, and let stand for 1 minute then cook for another 40 seconds, stir, and let stand for another minute. Check the oats are soft (if not, give it another 20 seconds on full).

Slice in the banana and allow to cool a little.

Stylish soup

Aah... soup. It's a hug in a bowl. There's nothing quite like cradling a steamy hot bowl of soup in ice-cold hands, aromas drifting nose-height from the kitchen. I just love soup. It can be any flavor you like, creamy, spicy or herby; it's nutritious, a substantial well-balanced meal, quick to prepare and—for the most culinary phobic among you—simple to make.

All you need is a chopping board, a knife, one huge pot, and away you go. Simply ladle it into big, generous bowls or mugs (no spoons required) or have it on the run in a large, portable thermos bottle.

And add a little extra liquid and your soup will streeettch to feed an army. That's exactly why soup was "invented" in the 1800s by an Anglo-American, Count Rumford. While in Bavaria he was in a stew trying to figure out how to keep his troops well nourished. "Soup," his "discovery," was as exciting as vaccinations or Franklin's lightning bolt. Soup was going to eradicate world hunger.

Count Rumford believed starches—potatoes and barley—would keep his men going for hours. So he threw these two ingredients into an enormous pot and for flavor he added a bucketful of legumes and onion and celery. Before serving, each bowl received a crowning of cheese, fish, or meat and a piece of stale bread. His men thrived and the idea spread throughout the armies of Europe. Soup went on to save the lives of thousands in the Great Depression when soup kitchens sprang up to feed the unemployed and destitute. And, even better, soup can save your bacon when you need it too.

Cheesy Broccoli, Cauliflower, and Potato Soup

Makes 1 serving

¹⁄₂ cup water	2 tablespoons mature
¹⁄₃ cup broccoli	cheddar, grated
¹⁄₃ cup cauliflower	¹⁄₂ cup whole milk
¹⁄₃ cup potato	Freshly ground black pepper
or 7 cubes of frozen Broccoli,	Small pinch of salt
Cauliflower, and Potato	
Purée (see page 87)	

Bring the water to a rolling boil. Wash and trim the broccoli and cauliflower. Wash and peel the potato, then finely hand chop or run through the grater attachment of a food processor—the fine chop will speed up the cooking time. Immediately pour the chopped mix into the boiling water and simmer for 5 minutes.

Add the cheese and stir in with the milk. Return to a simmer, season, and serve.

Corn Chowder

Makes 1 serving

2 teaspoons olive oil	Freshly ground black pepper
1/3 cup leek	Small pinch of salt
1/3 cup baby corn	(for a larger meal add 1/3 cup
1/4 cup peas (fresh or frozen)	chopped, cooked chicken or
1/3 cup potato	steamed, flaked white fish)
7 fl oz whole milk	
1/4 cup water	

Heat the olive oil in a medium saucepan. Finely slice the leek into thin disks and sweat in the olive oil to soften.

Rinse the baby corn and also slice into thin disks; add baby corn and peas to the leeks.

Wash and peel the potato, then cut into small cubes (approx. 1/4 inch). Add the potato, milk, and water and boil, then simmer for 10 minutes until the potato is soft.

If you prefer a thick smooth soup rather than chunky, blend with a hand blender (adding the optional fish or chicken). Season and serve.

Carrot, Sweet Potato, and Cilantro Soup

Makes 1 serving

2 teaspoons olive oil	1/2 cup water
1/4 medium onion	Freshly ground black pepper
2/3 cup carrot	Small pinch of salt
2/3 cup sweet potato	1 tablespoon freshly chopped
or 7 cubes of frozen Carrot	cilantro
and Sweet Potato Purée	
(see page 86)	
1/2 cup whole milk	

Heat the olive oil in a medium saucepan. Finely chop the onion and sauté until soft but not browned. Wash, peel, and finely chop or grate the carrot and sweet potato and sauté

for a further 2–3 minutes or add the frozen purée to defrost, stirring continuously.

Add the milk and water and bring to a simmer.

Liquidize with a hand blender, season, and add the cilantro. For an extra treat, swirl through a tablespoonful of crème fraîche.

Spicy Bean Soup

Makes 1 serving

1/4 onion	1 1/2 cups mixed beans
1 garlic clove	Pinch of cayenne pepper or
2 teaspoons olive oil	2–3 drops Tabasco
1 fresh tomato (or 1/2 canned	1 teaspoon Worcestershire
plum tomato)	sauce
1/2 inch cube of fresh ginger,	Freshly ground black pepper
peeled and grated or	Small pinch of salt
1/4 teaspoon dried ginger	1 teaspoon freshly chopped
1/2 cup tomato juice or 1/2 cup	chives
water and 1/2 tablespoon	
tomato paste	

Finely chop the onion and crush the garlic.

Heat the olive oil in a medium saucepan and sauté the onion and garlic until soft but not browned.

Chop the tomato and add to the pan with the finely grated ginger, and sauté for a further 2–3 minutes.

Add the tomato juice (or water and tomato paste). Rinse the beans and stir into the soup and season with the cayenne, Worcester sauce, pepper, and salt. Bring back to a boil.

Either liquidize with a hand blender or keep it chunky. Add the chives just before serving.

Salads

Hallelujah. Praise the lettuce. The salad just may be the answer to your nutritional prayers. For food in a flash it's easy to toss together a nutrient-packed salad. All you need is fresh ingredients, a big chopping board, a sharp knife, and a generously sized salad bowl.

Salads provide you with several of your 5-a-day requirements (remember one portion is equal to one medium fruit or a quarter of a cup of dried fruit). However, what the 5-a-day mantra doesn't stipulate is that you really need a color mix to get the right range of nutrients too (see A pot of nutritional gold, opposite). It also pays—health- and walletwise—to buy local vegetables and fruits in season. The closer you can eat your food to its natural, fresh-from-the-ground state the more nutritious it is likely to be—you don't want it suffering from food miles jetlag.

When you build your salad, think in terms of a food pyramid. Start with a base layer of fresh green leaves. Next, "eat with your eye": select an artful, Picasso-like mix of brightly colored vegetables and fruit. For a slow-releasing energy burn that will last all afternoon, choose a selection of low-GI foods, like boiled potatoes in their skins, whole-wheat pasta shells or cooked lentils. Crown your salad with a protein (think broiled chicken, ham, cheese, boiled egg, tuna fish, mackerel). The X-factor? Garnish with fresh herbs or toasted seeds.

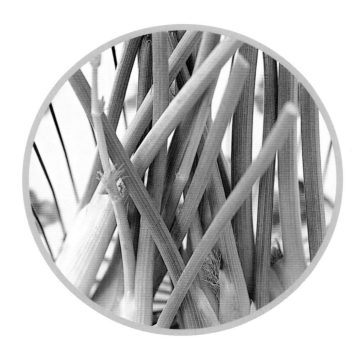

A pot of nutritional gold

When you choose a rainbow of vegetables and fruits, you get the right balance of vitamins and minerals as well as a range of antioxidants.

Go Green
Darker green in fruit and vegetables signifies extra goodness. Green vegetables and fruit contain chlorophyll, the plant's way of converting sunlight to energy. Greens have vitamins A, C, and E as well as a mix of minerals, but dark greens also contain lutein and indoles, which have antioxidant, health-promoting properties.
Sources: peas, broccoli, green peppers, cucumber, spinach, and asparagus.

See Red
The natural red blusher in fruit and vegetables are lycopene or anthocyanins, two antioxidants (these neutralize "free radicals" or unstable oxygen molecules that can damage cells).
Sources: watermelons, tomatoes, pink grapefruits, red potatoes, red cabbage, beets, cherries.

Bright Almighty
Orange and yellow fruit or vegetables are jam-packed full of natural pigments called carotenoids. Adults who eat plenty of vegetables high in carotenoids significantly reduce their chances of heart attack. Pumpkins, yams, sweet potatoes, and carrots are full of beta-carotene (vitamin A) while citrus fruits are full of vitamin C.
Sources: yellow peppers, oranges, apricots, peaches, yellow plums, corn.

Get the Blues
Purple and blue-hued vegetables and fruits are colored by water-soluble antioxidant pigments anthocyanins and phenolics, which may help to prevent cancer, stroke, and heart disease as well as improve our memories.
Sources: beets, blueberries, eggplants, grapes, raisins, figs, plums.

All White
White fruits and vegetables contain more "anthoxanthins" as well as health-promoting chemicals such as allicin, reputed to lower cholesterol and blood pressure and reduce risk of stomach cancer and heart disease.
Sources: bananas, cauliflower, garlic, parsnips, onions.

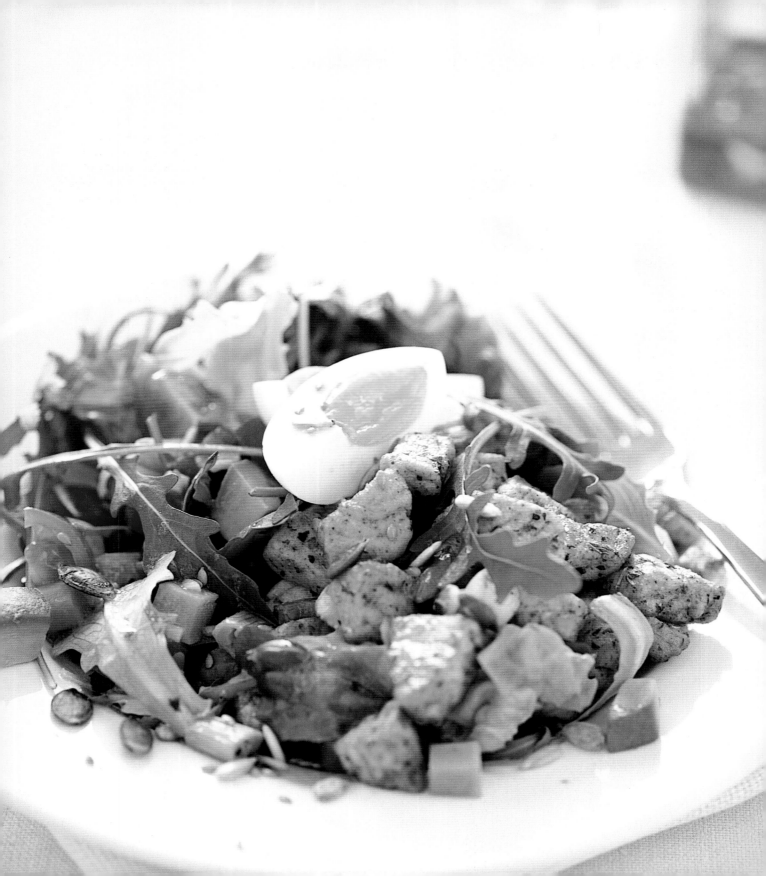

Salmon with Warm Wilted Salad

Makes 1–2 servings

¼ cup mixed kernals
(e.g. sunflower kernals,
pumpkin kernals)
1 egg
½ pound salmon
½ tablespoon olive oil
2–3 green onions
3 cups salad greens (e.g. baby
   spinach, arugula,
   watercress)
Choose from a selection of:
½ red pepper
1 small carrot
½ avocado

5–6 button mushrooms
1 small tomato or a few
   cherry tomatoes
TO COAT THE FISH
1 tablespoon wholewheat
   flour
1 teaspoon dried herbs
   (mixed or single, e.g.
   oregano, basil)
Pinch of salt
Fresh ground black pepper
Up to ¼ teaspoon spice of
   your choice (e.g. paprika,
   ginger, chilli)

Toast the kernals in a nonstick skillet (do not add oil, simply heat the pan and keep the kernals moving). Set aside. Hardboil the egg, about 5–6 minutes, and cool off in cold water (to prevent the yolk blackening).

On a dinner plate combine the ingredients for the coating. Wash and chop the fish into 2 inch squares. Roll the fish in the seasoned flour mix. Chop the vegetables into 1 inch pieces. Peel and quarter the egg.

Gently heat the olive oil in the nonstick skillet and pan fry the salmon for approximately 5 minutes on each side until golden. Chop the green onions into ½ inch pieces and add halfway through the cooking.

Meanwhile arrange the washed salad greens on a serving plate and sprinkle with your chosen vegetables.

Place the hot salmon and quartered egg on top of the salad.

Turn off the heat then pour the vinaigrette into the still warm pan and stir round to pick up the flavors of the fish and green onion. Pour over the salad to wilt the leaves. Finally top off with the toasted kernals.

Vinaigrette

Makes 2–3 servings

1 tablespoon olive oil
1 tablespoon freshly
   squeezed lemon juice or
   cider vinegar
Choose from a selection of:
1 garlic clove, crushed
1 teaspoon mild mustard, e.g.
   Dijon or wholegrain

2 drops of Tabasco or small
   pinch of mild chili powder
1 teaspoon fresh chopped
   herbs or pinch of dried herbs
Freshly ground black pepper

For best results, put all the ingredients in a lidded jar and shake. The dressing will keep for 2–3 days if chilled.

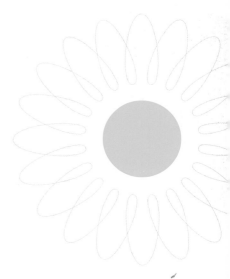

Sorted Caesar

The traditional Caesar Salad can be a simple combination of lettuce, tomato, parmesan, and croûtons with or without chicken. My Sorted Caesar adds a few extra ingredients to bring in a few more important colors, giving you a wider range of nutrients.

Makes 1 serving

1 slice mixed-grain bread	¼ avocado
½ tablespoon olive oil (optional)	2 anchovy fillets
	¼ yellow pepper
1 garlic clove (optional)	¼ red onion
2 cups Romaine or Iceberg leaves	½ cup cooked chicken breast
4–5 cherry tomatoes	2 tablespoons parmesan cheese

If you like croûtons cut the bread into cubes, heat the oil and garlic in a nonstick skillet, fry the cubes until golden and set aside to cool. If croûtons are not your thing, simply toast the bread and cut into cubes to give a little crunch to the salad.

Wash and tear the leaves and arrange in a bowl. Wash and slice the cherry tomatoes, avocado, anchovy, pepper and onion, then add to the leaves. Slice the cooked chicken (also works well with lightly smoked trout) and top with parmesan shavings and croûtons or toasted bread cubes.

Drizzle with Simple Caesar Salad Dressing (see below).

Simple Caesar Salad Dressing

Again—not quite the traditional… but quick and delicious.

2 teaspoons fresh lemon juice	1 garlic clove, crushed
2 teaspoons olive oil	Splash Worcestershire sauce
1 teaspoon Dijon mustard	1 tablespoon very finely grated parmesan cheese
1 teaspoon crème fraîche, natural yogurt or mayonnaise	Freshly ground black pepper
	Tiny pinch of salt

Combine all the ingredients in a lidded jar and shake.

Nuts About Cheese

Two brazil nuts contain an adult's daily requirement of selenium, an important mineral in creating uplifting and positive moods.

If you or your partner have a family history of nut allergies it would be advisable to avoid nuts and sesame seeds if breastfeeding. Sunflower, linseed and pumpkin kernals are known to be less allergenic.

Makes 1 serving

3–4 small salad potatoes	1 cup mixed salad greens
½ carrot	2 ounces goat's cheese
¼ cup snow peas	4–5 sun-dried tomatoes
¼ red pepper	¼ cup mixed nuts
2 green onions	

Wash and halve the potatoes and boil or steam until soft. Allow to cool.

Wash, peel, and slice the carrot. Wash and slice the snow peas, red pepper, and green onions. Arrange the chopped vegetables and potato on the salad greens.

Cut the goat's cheese into cubes and broil until lightly golden, place on the salad with the sun-dried tomatoes, and sprinkle with the nuts.

Drizzle with vinaigrette (see page 43).

Bakes

Bakes are great, all-in-one meals, ideal for making in batches then freezing. Defrost overnight in the fridge or on a low (defrost) setting in the microwave, then cover and heat through in the oven or microwave. Bakes are particularly warming in winter and fill the house with comforting homey aromas.

Lentil Bake

Makes 1–2 servings

1 tablespoon olive oil
1 small onion and/or leek
1–2 garlic cloves
1/3 cup mushrooms
1/2 medium sweet potato or
  squash (butternut is good)
1 medium carrot
1/3 cup broccoli
1/2 cup red lentils
2/3 cup water or water
  and milk
1–2 teaspoons fresh mixed
  herbs or 1/2–1 teaspoon

dried mixed herbs
1/4 cup sunflower, pumpkin
  and flax seeds (linseed)
Pinch of cayenne pepper
  (optional)
Freshly ground black pepper

FOR THE TOPPING
1–2 ounces whole-wheat or
  wholegrain bread
3 tablespoons hard cheese,
  grated (optional)

Preheat the oven to 400°F.

Lightly toast the bread for the topping and set aside to cool and harden. Heat the oil in a medium saucepan. Peel and roughly chop the onion and/or leek, slice the garlic (it gives a milder taste than crushing), and sauté in the oil for 2 minutes.

Wash, peel, and chop the other vegetables and add to the pan. Rinse the lentils and check over for any grit, then add to the pan. Stir, pour in the water and simmer for 10–15 minutes until the lentils soften but still have a little hardness, adding more water as needed. Add the herbs, kernals, and seasoning, then pour the mixture into an ovenproof dish.

Crumble the toast—either tear, chop, or chop briefly in a hand blender's chopping attachment—sprinkle on to the mix, and finish off with grated cheese. Bake for 25–30 minutes until the lentils are soft and the topping golden.

Shepherd's Pie

Makes 2–3 servings

1/4 pound ground meat
  (traditionally lamb,
  alternatively beef or turkey)
1 small onion
1/2 cup carrot
1 tablespoon peas (fresh or
  frozen) or broccoli
1 teaspoon mixed herbs e.g.
  mint, thyme, marjoram, basil
  (fresh or dried)
1/3 cup tomatoes
  (fresh or canned)
Dash of Worcestershire sauce

Freshly ground black pepper
  and small pinch of salt
  (optional)

FOR THE TOPPING
3/4 pound potatoes
1 tablespoon milk
2 teaspoons butter
Freshly ground black pepper
3 tablespoons grated cheese

Preheat the oven to 400°F.

Put the ground meat in a medium saucepan, add the chopped onion, and cook until the meat changes color from red to brown. Keep the mixture moving as it cooks; there is likely to be enough fat in the meat without adding any oil, but if it sticks add a little drizzle of olive oil.

Wash, peel, and cube or grate the carrot into the mixture and stir in the peas and herbs. Chop the tomatoes and stir into the pan with the seasoning, and gently simmer.

Wash, peel, and cube the potatoes—smaller cubes will cook faster. Bring a pan of water to a boil, add the potatoes, and simmer or steam until soft. Mash with the milk, butter, and pepper.

Spoon the meat mixture into an ovenproof dish, then layer on the potatoes, and finally top with grated cheese. Bake for 30–35 minutes until the cheese bubbles and begins to brown.

Three-Fish Bake

Makes 1 large bake or 2 single bakes

1 egg	$1/4$ **pound salmon**
1 pound sweet potato	$1/4$ **pound white fish**
1$1/2$ tablespoons olive oil	$1/4$ **pound smoked or fresh**
1 garlic clove, crushed	**mackerel**
(optional)	1 heaped teaspoon cornstarch
1 leek, trimmed or 1 medium	1 cup milk
onion	Salt and pepper
1 medium carrot	A few sprigs of dill
$1/2$ green pepper	1 cup broccoli florets
1 teaspoon chopped capers	4 tablespoons grated cheese

Preheat the oven to 400°F.

Hardboil the egg (about 6–7 minutes). Peel and chop the sweet potato. Bring a large pan of water to a boil, add the potato, and simmer for 10–15 minutes until the potato has softened. Drain, mash, and set aside.

Place $1/4$ tablespoon olive oil and garlic, if using, in the bottom of two single-serving round ovenproof dishes or $1/2$ tablespoon olive oil in one larger round ovenproof pie dish. Heat the remaining olive oil in a large frying pan. Chop the leek and sauté. Peel and chop the carrot, dice the pepper and add to the leek with the capers. Gently cook for 5 minutes.

Skin the fish if you prefer, chop into $1/4$ inch chunks, then chop the boiled egg and add to the frying pan.

Mix the cornstarch with a little milk to form a smooth paste then add the rest of the milk. Pour over the fish and vegetable mixture and stir through. Season with pepper, a small pinch of salt, and most of the dill (keep a little to garnish). Cover, bring to a boil, and simmer, stirring occasionally.

Divide the mixture between the two dishes or put it all in the larger dish. Arrange the broccoli on top and dollop the mashed sweet potato between the florets. Sprinkle the cheese on top.

Bake in the oven for 20 minutes until the topping begins to brown.

If you have made two bakes, enjoy one bake now and allow the other to cool, then freeze. Once frozen, you may find that you can release the bake from its dish and place in a freezer bag, thus freeing up the dish for another baking day.

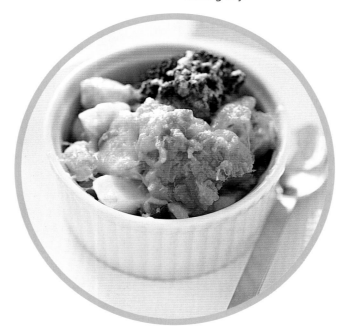

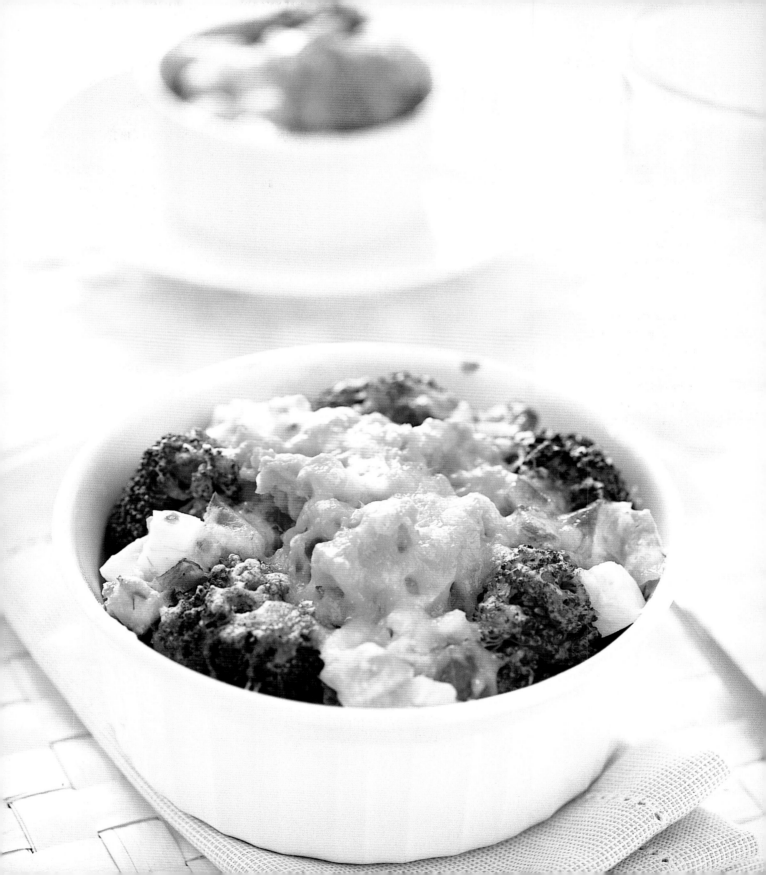

Quick fixes

Are you ready to bite somebody's head off? Dealing with small children is always going to be more *Amityville Horror* than *The Sound of Music* when your system is out of whack. So, stop, get yourself into the kitchen, and follow some of the quick-and-easy recipes below. Simply mix up one of the suggested toppings and use on a base of potatoes, egg noodles, whole wheat spaghetti or squash it in between two bits of fresh bread or into a pita pocket. Your children will notice the change from Frankenstein's monster to Mother Teresa almost immediately.

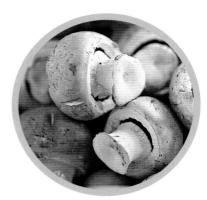

Creamy Salmon and Dill

Makes 2 servings

¹/₄ pound salmon
2 tablespoons crème fraîche
Juice of ¹/₂ lemon
1 teaspoon capers (optional)
2 teaspoons freshly chopped dill

Freshly ground black pepper
Pinch of salt
A few spinach or mixed salad greens

Steam the fish for 6–8 minutes until it is cooked through. Flake and allow to cool.

Combine the fish, crème fraîche, lemon juice, chopped capers, if using, and dill with a good pinch of fresh ground black pepper and a little salt.

Use with the salad greens to top a baked potato, add crunch to a sandwich, or you could wilt the leaves by stirring the mix through hot pasta.

Mediterranean Moment

Makes 1 serving

¹/₂ cup red, green and yellow peppers
2–3 button mushrooms
¹/₄ zucchini
¹/₂ tablespoon olive oil
1 garlic clove, crushed
¹/₂ cup buffalo mozzarella, chopped

1 ounce sun-dried tomatoes
1 ounce olives, pitted
1 teaspoon fresh oregano and basil or ¹/₄–¹/₂ teaspoon dried Italian mixed herbs
1 teaspoon pesto
Freshly ground black pepper

Chop and combine the ingredients (leave out the garlic if you prefer) with a little vinaigrette (see page 43).

Or, heat a ridged griddle (or nonstick skillet). Chop the peppers, mushrooms, and zucchini and toss in the olive oil and crushed garlic. Chargrill and remove from the heat.

Sprinkle with the chopped mozzarella, sun-dried tomatoes, olives, herbs, and stir in the pesto. Season with pepper. This is a great filling for Italian flat bread or baked potato. It also works very well stirred through hot or cold pasta.

Va Va Voom

Makes 1 serving

1–2 teaspoons toasted
  linseed, sunflower, and
  pumpkin kernals
¼ cup cream cheese or
  cottage cheese

½ small red onion or
  1–2 green onions
½ beef tomato
1 cup spinach or salad greens
Freshly ground black pepper

Toast the kernals in a dry nonstick skillet (keep them moving to prevent them burning). If time is really short, then simply use untoasted.

Stir the kernals into the cheese. Slice the onion and tomato. Wash the greens.

Layer the ingredients on to a mixed-grain bun, or a baked sweet potato. Season and serve.

Zesty Tuna

Makes 1 serving

¼ cup snow peas
¼ cup baby corn
1 small tomato
⅓ cup cooked fresh tuna (or
  canned tuna in water)
¼ unwaxed lemon
1 tablespoon natural yogurt

A few fresh basil leaves
3 tablespoons cheddar
  cheese, grated (Optional.
  You may choose to use less
  tuna if adding cheese.)
Freshly ground black pepper

Wash and slice the snow peas, baby corn, and tomato.

Flake the tuna, zest the lemon, and combine with the yogurt.

Layer the tuna mixture, baby corn, snow peas, tomato, basil, and grated cheese on to fresh bread, baked potato, or cold pasta. Season with black pepper.

In colder weather use the mixture as a filling for a whole-wheat pita pocket and broil for 3 minutes.

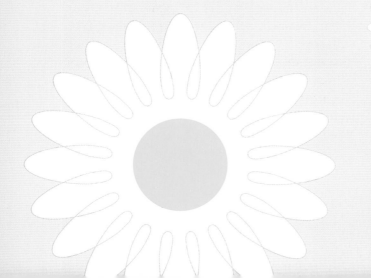

Desserts

Watch your step here because desserts can dazzle you with calories and leave you with little nutrition. Others will take you to the heights of ecstasy only to dump you when they run out of energy. So it's important you're seduced by healthy types who will give you the world of vitamins and minerals. Take, for example, the nicely presented fresh fruit salad. A safe, reliable choice and if you devour a vitamin-C-rich salad after an iron-rich meal you'll maximize your iron uptake—and give yourself more energy.

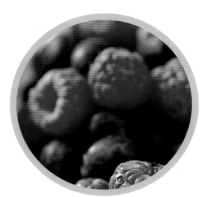

The way to your nutritional heart should be via a dessert without the sugar daddy sweeteners. Fruit should provide all the sweetness you need. What's more, don't be afraid to let a good-looking, nutrient-laden dessert join you for a great breakfast. An oaty crumble first thing in the morning, heated up from the leftovers of the night before should put a spring in your step for the rest of the day.

You shouldn't have to make something new each time; simply make more than you need and freeze the rest. For example, when you're making a crumble, cook the apples, pears, or mango, then freeze a helping to make a base for a crumble in the future. If your baby is coming up to weaning, double your quantities and make single purées for them and grown-up combos for yourself.

Fruit Salad

This is not so much a recipe as a reminder—when choosing fruit, keep the "Pot of gold" idea for a savory salad in your mind (see page 41). Keep a multicolored fruit bowl on the go and aim for a lidded container of diced fruit salad in the fridge to scoop into breakfast, snack with yogurt, or serve as dessert. Liven things up with fresh herbs, such as mint and cilantro, and be adventurous—strawberries, for example, are delicious with black pepper and balsamic vinegar.

Oaty Crumble

Makes 2–3 servings

1 cup fruit, e.g. apples, pears, rhubarb, gooseberries, golden raisins	FOR THE CRUMBLE
	2 tablespoons butter
	3 tablespoons whole-wheat flour
¼ teaspoon of spice, e.g. cinnamon, ginger	1 teaspoon brown sugar
1 teaspoon brown sugar (optional)	½ cup oats
	2 tablespoons mixed kernals, e.g. sunflower, linseeds

Wash and chop the fruit and gently simmer with the spice and sugar, if using, in 1 tablespoon of water until they start to soften (if you like the fruit to have a little bite you could miss out this stage).

Preheat the oven to 400°F. Arrange the fruit in a small ovenproof bowl.

To make the crumble, grate the butter into the flour and sugar in a medium mixing bowl and rub in until the mixture resembles breadcrumbs. Stir in the oats and kernals.

Top the fruit with the crumble and bake for 25 minutes or until the crumble begins to brown.

Why not try a tropical crumble? Choose mango, pineapple, and banana to make an exotic base, then add coconut flakes and Brazil nuts into the topping.

Baked Apple

Grandma Daisy—the inspiration behind my company name—had apple and plum trees in her garden so baked fruits were a regular treat. Around Christmastime the filling was switched from the dried fruit stuffing in this recipe to homemade mincemeat—delicious but also incredibly quick and easy. This also works with a large pear.
Makes 1 serving

1 teaspoon currants, golden
  raisins or raisins
2 dried apricots (pitted)
2 ready-to eat-prunes or dates
  (pitted)
Juice of 1/4 lemon
1 teaspoon kernels or nuts
  (omit if adapting this recipe
  for a child)

1 cooking apple or large
  eating apple (if using
  cooking apple add 1
  teaspoon brown sugar)
1 tablespoon butter

Preheat the oven to 400°F.

Combine the dried fruit, lemon juice, and kernals (and nuts and sugar if using) in the chopping attachment of a hand blender and coarsely chop with a quick blitz.

Wash the apple but do not peel. Use a corer to remove the core—you may wish to core out a little more to fit in more filling. Use a sharp knife and score an incision around the middle of the apple, making sure that you cut through the skin but not deep enough to cut through to the hole at the base. Place the apple in a small ovenproof dish or mini baking tray.

Push the dried fruit into the hole then top up with the butter—don't worry if there isn't enough room, the melting butter will coat the top of the apple, helping it to go slightly crisp and golden. Bake for 20–30 minutes until you can push a sharp knife easily into the fruit and the top is golden. Serve hot, with a blob of yogurt or crème fraîche if you like.

(Avoid nuts, particularly peanuts, if you or your partner have a family history of nut allergy.)

Baked Banana

OK—we all like chocolate—this ultra-simple recipe combines a way to get one of the 5 fruits a day with a bit of indulgence—and if you choose quality (+70 percent cocoa solid), organic chocolate you will get a mood enhancing dose of endorphins and serotonin, not just a crash-and-burn sugar hit of lower-quality confectionery.
Makes 1 serving

1 banana

4–5 chunks chocolate

Preheat the oven to 350°F.

Don't peel the banana, just use a sharp knife to slice a slit lengthwise and slot in the chocolate chunks. Wrap in foil and bake for 20 minutes.

Granita

You'll be making lots of delicious fruit purées for your baby in the next few months—if you have time to make some early, freeze a few cubes then use the rest to treat yourself and your partner to a fancy granita.
Makes 1 serving

1/2 cup fruit purée from stage
  1 or 2 (avoid banana and
  other fruits that don't freeze
  well)

Add spices of your choice, e.g.
  cinnamon, cardamom

Pour the purée into a freezable container with a lid. Part freeze for 30–40 minutes to a slush then whisk it up with a fork, repeat the freezing and forking one or two more times until you have fruit ice grains.

Serve in a decorative glass with a sprig of fresh mint.

Stage one:
First steps in weaning

Your child's first encounter with rice, fruit, and vegetables. A guide to great first-stage purées and when to introduce them into your baby's diet.

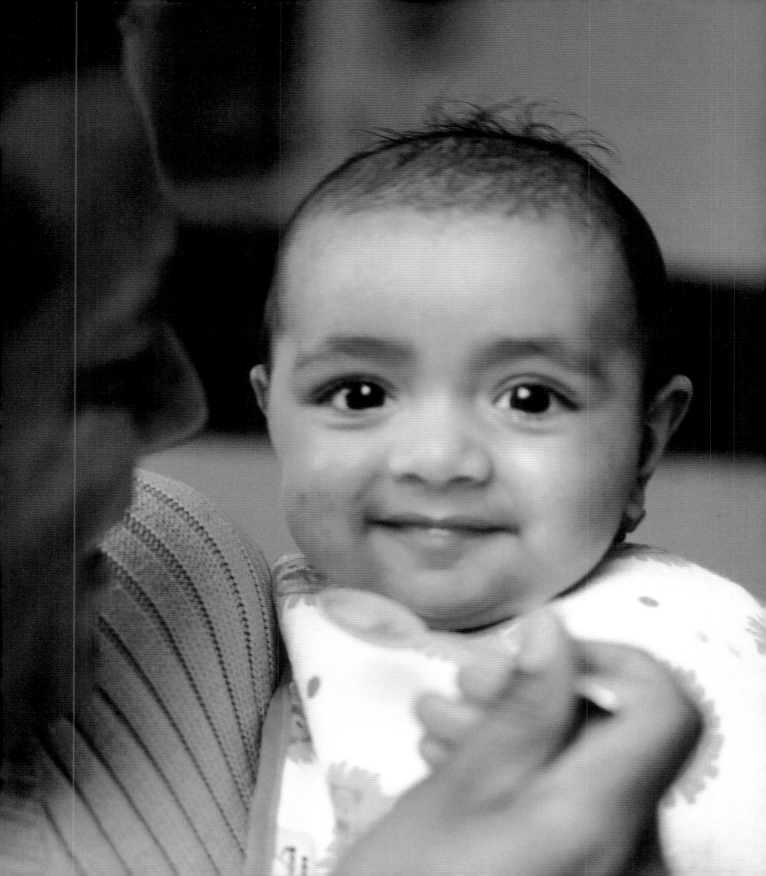

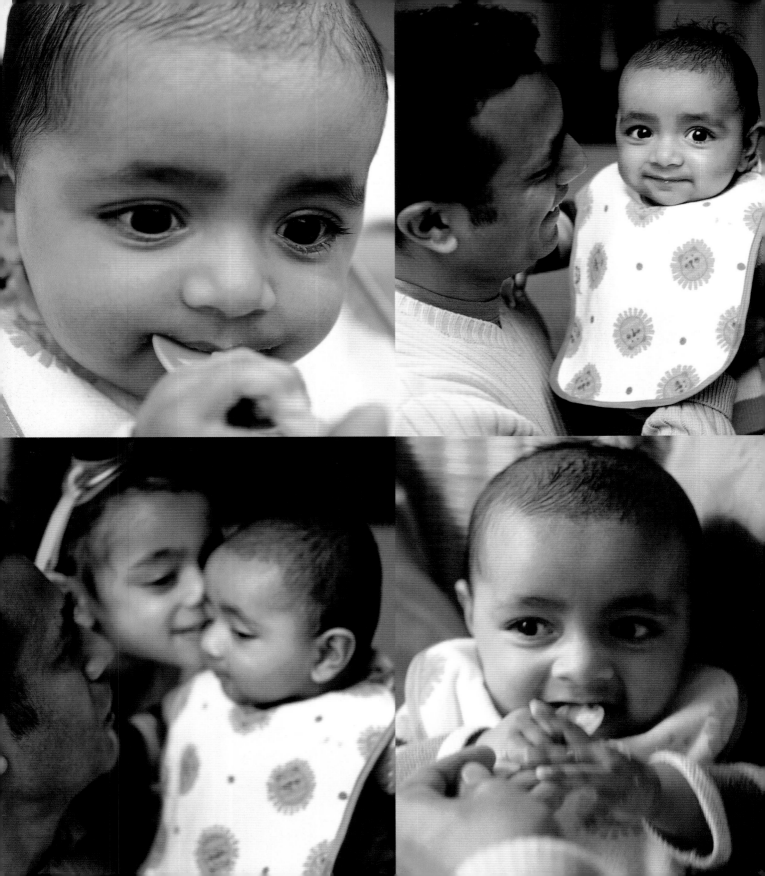

The first stage

How can you tell when your baby is ready for weaning? Your baby will let you know (for more, see the panel on page 56). There's no magic age or weight, but there are physical, emotional, and nutritional yardsticks that will indicate it's time to let the puréeing begin.

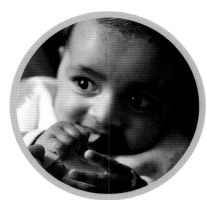

Like us, all babies are individuals. The key is not to start too soon or too late. Mothers of small babies particularly are often pressured into weaning too early, but the fact is a teaspoon of breast or formula milk contains more calories than a teaspoon of carrots.

Can I wean too soon?

Introducing food too early means that babies run the risk of developing food allergies and intolerances. Why? From birth to 4–6 months of age, babies have what's known as an "open gut," which means that the spaces between the cells of the small intestines allow food molecules, including whole proteins, to pass directly into the bloodstream. While this is great news for beneficial antibodies in breast milk, it also means that large proteins from other potentially allergy-forming foods can go right through, too. Babies start producing their own antibodies at about 6 months, when the gut "closes."

It takes up to 4 months for the lining of the baby's gut to develop and the kidneys to mature enough to cope with the waste products from solid food. If solids are introduced before a baby has a complete set of enzymes required to digest food properly, their digestive system could be damaged. Some digestive enzymes (like gastin and pepsin) reach adult levels around 3–4 months, while starch-busting and carbohydrate-crunching enzymes reach adult levels at around 6 months. Babies have low levels of lipase and bile salts, so fat digestion isn't even considered until around 6 months. Babies are born with a store of iron; however, by 6 months most babies have used up their iron reserves and even if they are drinking iron-fortified milk, it's important to include iron-rich foods.

Even before you start to wean your baby you can get them interested in mealtimes by sitting them with the family. And, yes, they can have their very own breast milk, formula, or cooled boiled water. Give your baby spoons, cups, bowls, and other utensils to play with or make your own "moms-icle" (a popsicle made from breast or formula milk).

Do I have to wait 6 months?

You may be aware of the World Health Organization's guidelines on when to wean. Initially they stated babies should be breastfed exclusively until 6 months. More recent recommendations have been clarified: Weaning should NOT be earlier than 4 months. The introduction of simple fruit and vegetable purées prior to 6 months is only acceptable if the baby is showing the signs of being ready to wean (see panel on page 56).

During the first months of weaning, your baby will need both first-stage purées and breast or formula milk.

I welcome these guidelines as it is all about when your baby is ready and not when the calendar dictates. If you are in any doubt seek the advice of your pediatrician.

The psychology of weaning

One of the most important things to remember when you start feeding your baby is your attitude. What you think of foods—your own conditioning—is easily passed on to your baby. Many of us get a glint in our eye when we talk about cake or chocolate, so it's no wonder our children grow up thinking these foods are desirable. Likewise, if we show limited enthusiasm for, say, cauliflower or Brussels sprouts (what is it about sprouts?), when we serve them to our children they get the idea these foods aren't attractive. What you communicate to your child conditions their attitude, so say, "Oh—delicious—try this tasty sprout," or, "Yummy body-building broccoli."

Tongue-thrust reflex

Your baby has all sorts of innate survival mechanisms, which is why, for example, you can take your baby swimming as your little Thorpedo knows instinctively not to breathe under water. Well, here's another to marvel at. Babies who are too young to wean will poke their tongue out if you try to give them solids too soon. This reflex stops them from choking by clearing the throat and mouth. So if your baby is poking their tongue out at you they aren't being cheeky, they are telling you it's too soon for purées.

Avoiding allergies

A food allergy occurs when your immune system tries to protect you unnecessarily against something you've eaten. It produces antibodies it would normally generate to protect itself from infection. The body goes into overdrive producing histamine and prostaglandins, which cause swelling and a possible drop in blood pressure almost immediately after eating the offending food, resulting in some or all of the symptoms shown opposite.

How common are allergic reactions?

Food allergies and intolerances get a lot of press and there is a general belief that they are on the increase, but this could be simply because we are becoming better at detecting

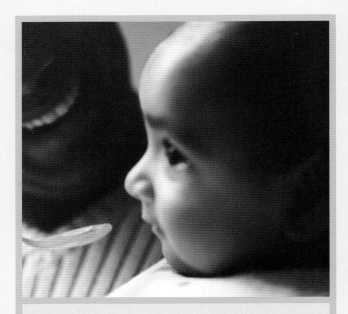

If your baby is at least 4 months old and shows these signs, it's time to get a hand blender

They're sitting up well without support

They're developing a "pincer" grasp

They're starting to demand feeds more often

They've lost the tongue-thrust reflex and don't automatically push solids out of their mouth

They're an eager mealtime participant and eye your food

They're ready and willing to chew

They used to sleep through the night but are now waking up

them. I believe that keeping food simple and, where possible, making it yourself to avoid the additives used by many manufacturers can help reduce the risk. During weaning, babies should not be given foods known to cause allergies, e.g. cow's milk, peanuts, eggs, soy, and tree nuts (walnuts, pecans, etc.) and gluten-rich foods, especially wheat. Other allergenic foods include pork, fish, and shellfish, oranges and citrus fruits, corn, berries, chocolate, tomatoes, and food additives.

Introduce new foods as single-variety purées at or before lunchtime. Try one at a time so you can clearly identify any trouble as well as likes and dislikes. This is particularly advisable where there is a family history of food allergies.

What to do in the event of an allergic reaction

If the reaction is extreme, e.g. fainting, difficulty in breathing, swelling of the eyes, lips or tongue or there is

Allergic reactions

Breathing problems

Swelling of the lips, eyes, or tongue

An increase in vomiting

Fainting

Bloating and excessive gas or diarrhea

Skin rashes and hives

Blistering in or around the mouth

Symptoms of food intolerance

Skin rashes including eczema and hives

Bloating and excessive gas or diarrhea

Ear infections or asthma

A runny nose and cold-like symptoms

Red, puffy eyes and eyelids, including dark circles under the eyes

Trouble sleeping, unexplained discomfort

instantaneous vomiting, call for an ambulance or take your child to the hospital immediately. Until you get help, check there is no object causing choking and loosen clothing around the neck and waist.

If you are worried about this, particularly if you or your partner have a family history of food allergies, ask your pediatrician for more information on one of the many excellent courses on first aid for your infant.

Food intolerance

Food intolerance can have symptoms similar to an allergy but doesn't involve antibodies. They rarely happen immediately and are often temporary—your child can grow out of them. The delayed reaction makes it difficult to work out the cause of the problem, but ongoing signs listed in the box on the left need to be investigated.

Getting started

Your baby is ready to be weaned, so it's time for a sumptuous serving of, er, baby rice. Mixed with baby's usual milk, it has a similar taste, but a slightly thicker texture. It's easy on the gut and has a low intolerance level. At this stage, milk is still the most important food. Solids are just first tastes and fillers, which should be introduced slowly over several weeks. Give your baby at least a third of their milk feed first. Then feed them some purée and finish with the rest of their milk feed. If your baby is drinking excessive amounts of milk and turning up their nose at solids, cut back on the lunchtime milk feed to stimulate the appetite.

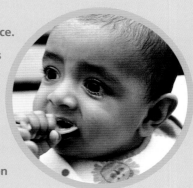

Ready

Offer a 1/4 teaspoon of cooked, warm baby rice on the tip of a shallow plastic spoon (metal ones can get too hot). If your baby doesn't like the taste and texture of the spoon, try putting the food on your (clean) finger and letting them suck it off. The best time of day to start is usually during the mid-morning or lunchtime feed as babies are less fussy then. This also gives you the rest of the day to keep an eye out for any reactions. After a couple of days, try a thin, runny single-ingredient vegetable puree, about the same kind of thickness as light cream. And, if this goes down well, repeat for a day or two; then it's time for another vegetable or fruit purée. Gradually make the purées a thicker consistency and try a little mixing.

Steady

If you walk down the supermarket aisle, you will see an exotic array of adult-sounding items, supposedly suitable as first weaning foods. Compared to a simple carrot purée they may sound exciting, but remember that for the first few months of life your baby has suckled away on just one food, milk. So far from boring, the bright color, subtle texture variation, and pure taste is an adventure in itself. Learning something new will require concentration and contemplation, so prepare to be patient.

Cook

Whether you intend to pan cook or steam, it's important to chop the ingredients into small uniform chunks so they're all ready at the same time. At Fresh Daisy, we chop ours up into 1/8 inch cubes. If you overcook the purée, it will lose its taste and texture. As a rule of thumb, most foods won't take more than 10 minutes. Try to use as little water as possible because vitamins such as B and C leech out into the water. If you plan to pan cook instead of steaming, the important thing is to add the fruit or vegetables to a pan of water already at a rolling boil. Where possible, add the vegetable water to the food processor to loosen up the purée and preserve the vitamins.

Alternatively, you could steam your vegetables and fruit, which is a better way of preserving the nutrients. Remember to use the collected stock from the steamer tray as part of the purée.

If you want to microwave the food, chop into small uniform chunks, put in a microwave friendly dish and just cover with water. Leave an air vent and cook on full power according to weight. Make sure you check and recheck the temperature of the purée since microwaves are notorious for cooking produce unevenly, and microwaved food is particularly prone to hot spots. Always stir thoroughly and check the food before offering to your baby.

Feed time

Look them in the eye and be enthusiastic about their eating. It's deeeelicious food and they're a wonnnnderful eater (even if the kitchen begins to look like Jackson Pollock's been visiting).

So, they like food. What do you do next? Gradually increase the number of solid food feeds from one to two then three a day, slowly increasing the portions of solid food to match your baby's appetite.

Over the next couple of weeks, introduce a new vegetable or fruit every second day, so they've had a wide variety. Variety is the spice of life, and as you'll read later there's evidence to suggest that a wide spectrum of tastes will help keep a 1-year-old open-minded about food.

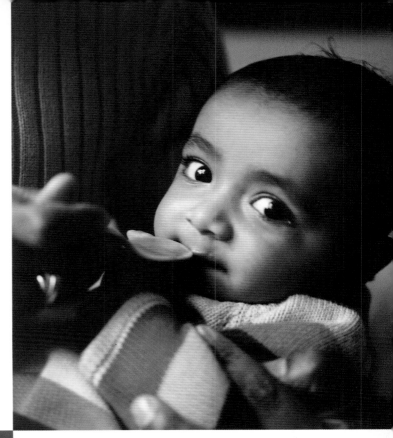

Baby rice

This is a great first weaning food. Once mixed with breast or formula milk, it seems just like thickened milk. It's bland and soft on your baby's immature digestive system and, later on, can also be an excellent food to relieve tummy upsets and diarrhea. Rice is also gluten-free (gluten can be an allergen and is found in cereals, wheat, rye, oats, and barley). You can use baby rice to thicken fruit (like pears) or vegetable purées, making them more filling.

The most convenient way to buy it is to get off-the-shelf packs from your local organic store. Simply follow the instructions on the pack.

Vegetable purées

I've tried to give you an idea of the number of servings you can expect from each recipe since the first time you try your baby on a new food. You may only need a teaspoonful so I've kept the measurements pretty small so you're not swimming in purée. Once you know that your baby likes a particular variety, multiply the quantities up and freeze batches in ice cube trays or small plastic pots.

Sweet Potato Purée

Sweet potatoes have a nutritional soulmate in the squash family. Like the squashes, they also carry vitamin D for healthy bones and vitamin E for immune systems. The orangey ones are better for your baby than the creamy colors since these contain beta-carotene or vitamin A. They also rate well on the potassium, vitamin C, and fiber stakes and contain vitamin B[3] or niacin, which helps to balance moods. As they're sweet with a high water content, they make an appetizing first food for tiny tastebuds.
Makes 1–3 servings

1 sweet potato (approx. ¼ pound)

Wash and peel, then grate or finely hand chop the sweet potato to around ⅛ inch dice. The finer you chop, the easier you'll find achieving a very smooth purée.

For the best results, steam for 10 minutes in an electric steamer. Alternatively in a small saucepan, bring just enough water to cover the sweet potato to a rolling boil, add the sweet potato and simmer for 10 minutes until the largest piece is soft. If you have the oven on anyway, just give a sweet potato a scrub down, stab it all over with a fork, and bake it for about 40 minutes at 300°F.

Scoop out the flesh and purée, using the chopping attachment of a hand blender, until smooth, adding a little boiled water if needed to create a glossy finish.

Finally push through a fine strainer or finest-grade food mill disk.

Carrot Purée

Carrots are a perfect weaning food for beginner foodies and are an excellent source of beta-carotene, which converts in the body to vitamin A, essential for good eyesight and skin. Beta-carotene also bolsters baby's immune system and acts as an antioxidant. The darker a carrot is, the more beta-carotene it contains, so choose older carrots over baby ones. The fiber in carrots also helps your baby's gut to eliminate foods smoothly. When baby is over 6 months, add a little olive oil since the body absorbs these nutrients better with fat.

Carrots are particularly susceptible to chemicals in the soil, so even if you are still skeptical about organic at least go the extra mile here.
Makes 1–3 servings

1 medium carrot

Wash, peel, and grate or chop the carrot as per the sweet potato (left).

Steam for 10 minutes in an electric steamer. Or bring just enough water to cover the carrot to a rolling boil, add the carrot, and simmer for 10 minutes until the largest piece is soft.

Purée, using the chopping attachment of a hand blender, until smooth, adding the carrot stock collected in the steamer tray to create a glossy finish.

Finally push through a fine strainer or finest-grade food mill disk.

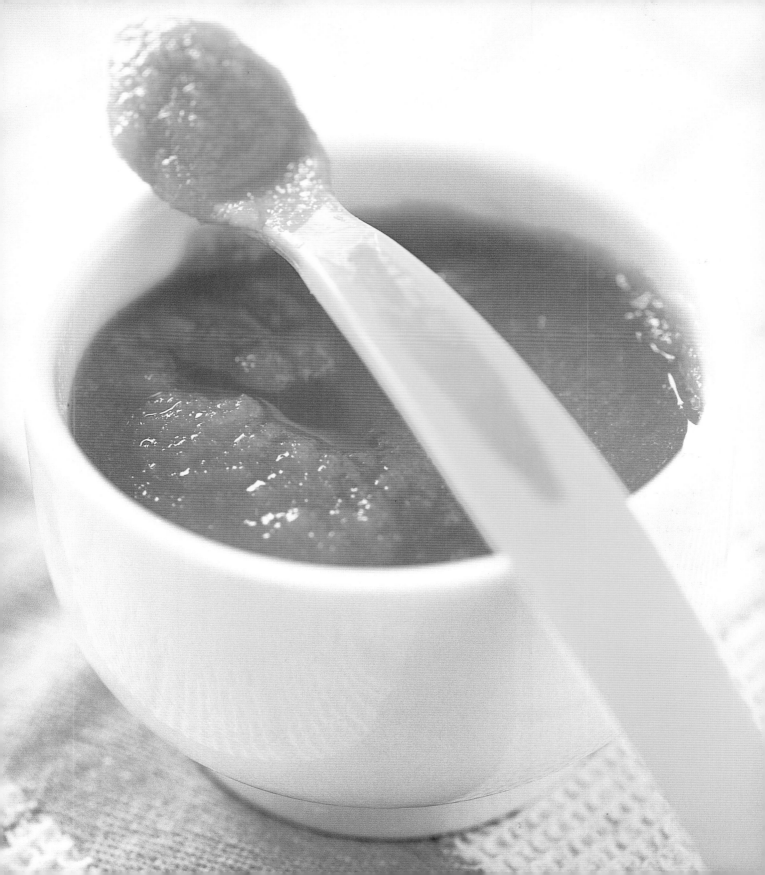

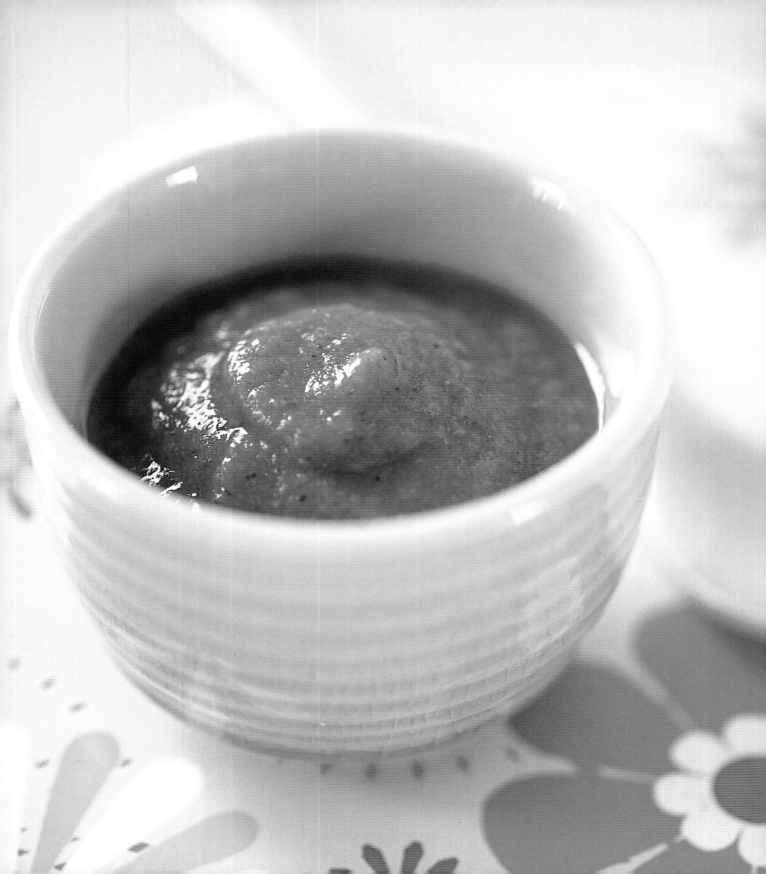

Broccoli Purée

This "structured" vegetable transcends the word "superfood" and almost demands a super-dooper league of its own. This one vegetable has so much goodness. For a start, it contains vitamin K, which helps blood coagulate and strengthens bones. It's also a rich source of magnesium and—get this—one raw serving has even more calcium than a pint of milk. It's an abundant source of vitamins B and C, too. Eaten regularly, one of broccoli's nutrients, glucosinolate, can help to prevent cancer. Broccoli has antibiotic and antiviral properties so will aid your baby to stay on top of the onslaught of childhood illnesses.
Makes 1–3 servings

1 cup broccoli

Wash and, especially with organic produce, check for bugs; there will be nothing dangerous—it's just a good sign the vegetable hasn't been sprayed with chemicals.

Put the florets through the grater attachment of a food processor or hand chop extremely finely—this will help the broccoli to cook through quickly. If you keep it as whole florets you will find you have to cook it for much longer to make the stems soft and you will lose taste and nutrients.

Steam for 8–10 minutes until the largest piece is soft. Broccoli is best steamed, but if you want to pan cook, bring 3–4 tablespoons of water to a rolling boil, then add the broccoli.

Purée, using the chopping attachment of a hand blender, until smooth, adding the broccoli stock collected in the steamer tray to create a glossy finish.

Finally push through a fine strainer or finest-grade food mill disk.

Cauliflower Purée

Cauliflower has a similar lineage to broccoli and possesses many of the same nutritional qualities as its high-flying cousin; however, like its color, cauliflower's nutritional achievements pale slightly beside those of its exceptional relative. Cauliflower possesses strong vitamin C as well as folic acid. A word of intestinal caution, however: while cauliflower's fibers will get your baby's intestinal tract working, it can make your baby burpy. Start introducing a little at a time.
Makes 1–3 servings

1 cup cauliflower

Cauliflower is delicious steamed. As with broccoli, wash and, especially with organic produce, check for bugs.

Put the florets through the grater attachment of a food processor or hand chop extremely finely to reduce the cooking time needed.

Steam for 8–10 minutes until the largest piece is soft. Or pan cook in a saucepan with enough boiling water to cover the cauliflower. Purée, using the chopping attachment of a hand blender, until smooth, adding the cauliflower stock collected in the steamer tray to create a glossy finish.

Finally push through a fine strainer or finest-grade food mill disk.

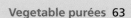

Butternut Squash Purée

Butternut squash makes more than just a good ghoul at Halloween. As an orange-colored vegetable, it—like carrot and sweet potato—is full of beta-carotene and vitamin C, an infection-busting duo. Other goodies include iron for carrying nutrients around the body and bone-building calcium and magnesium. Butternut squash also appeals to a baby's sweet palate, particularly after it's been baked in the oven, which gives it a slight caramel flavor. Mmm.
Makes 1–3 servings

⅔ cup butternut squash

Peel and remove any seeds and finely chop or grate the squash.

Steam or pan cook in 1–2 tablespoons of boiling water for 10–12 minutes until very soft.

Purée, using the chopping attachment of a hand blender, until smooth, adding the stock collected in the steamer tray or pan to create a glossy finish.

Finally push through a fine strainer or finest-grade food mill disk.

Alternatively, remove the seeds and wrap in foil (if you are doing a larger batch keep each chunk to about ⅔ cup and bake at 300°F for around 40 minutes or until soft. Scoop the soft flesh from the skin into the chopping bowl of your blender and continue as before. If needed, add a little boiling water to blend and push through a strainer as before.

Rutabaga Purée

The rutabaga is our name for the root vegetable originating from Sweden, called the *rotabagge*, and is closely related to the cabbage and, funnily enough, the turnip. Rutabagas are usually purple, white, or yellow in color, while the flesh should be white or a pale yellow. Like sweet potatoes and squash the vegetable is sweet to taste and makes a great stage 1 purée. Choose ones that are smooth, firm, and heavy. Rutabagas should be kept in the fridge and should last for about two weeks.
Makes 1–3 servings

⅔ cup rutabaga

Wash and peel, then grate or finely hand chop the rutabaga into ⅛ inch dice. The finer you chop, the easier you'll find achieving a very smooth purée.

Steam for 10 minutes in an electric steamer or bring just enough water to cover the swede to a rolling boil, add the swede, and simmer for 10 minutes until the largest piece is soft.

Purée, using the chopping attachment of a hand blender, until smooth, adding the stock collected in the steamer tray to create a glossy finish.

Finally push through a fine strainer or finest-grade food mill disk.

Parsnip Purée

Babies love parsnips. Like other root vegetables, these tend to be sweet. As well as iron, parsnips are rich in potassium, which is essential for the smooth functioning of muscles and nerves and also works to help the body absorb bone-growing calcium. On the vitamin front, they contain vitamins C and E as well as iron.
Makes 1–3 servings

1 parsnip (approx. ²⁄₃ cup)

Wash and peel, then grate or finely hand chop the parsnip into 1/8 inch dice. You may need to remove the core since this can harden while cooking and then you'll struggle to get it to purée.

For best results, steam for 10 minutes in an electric steamer. Alternatively, in a small saucepan add just enough water to cover the grated parsnip, bring to a boil, add the parsnip, and simmer for 10 minutes until the largest piece is soft.

Purée, using the chopping attachment of a hand blender, until smooth, adding the stock collected in the steamer tray to create a glossy finish.

Finally push through a fine strainer or finest-grade food mill disk.

If your baby finds the flavor of parsnip too strong, try mixing in a little apple or pear purée.

Pea Purée

It's a bird, it's a plane… it's super peas. Yes, these little balls are in the big nutrient league and considered an entire food in their own right. Peas have a vitamin and mineral punch of vitamins A, B, and C, zinc, magnesium, iron, and calcium. The little pea will help your baby's immune system as well as keep their bones growing and help their brains function. Frozen peas are perfectly fine: Just make sure they are used up within their freezer time and look out for supermarket varieties that are frozen on the day they are picked.
Makes 1–3 servings

¾ cup fresh or frozen peas

For best results, steam for 10 minutes in an electric steamer. Alternatively, in a small saucepan add just enough water to cover the peas, bring to a boil, add the peas, and simmer for 8—10 minutes until soft. Purée, using the chopping attachment of a hand blender, until smooth, adding the stock collected in the steamer tray to create a glossy finish.

Finally push through a fine strainer or finest-grade food mill disk to remove any stubborn pea skins.

Fennel Purée

Fennel may not be at the top of a list of weaning foods but you may want to consider it, especially with a baby who is suffering from colic. Weaning a baby too early increases the chances of colic and, although its causes are not completely understood, with your baby screaming the house down you'll know they have it. Overactive bowel contractions may be the problem and this, combined with trapped wind, is a recipe for an extremely unpleasant time. Fennel makes a pale green fragrant purée and is believed to have a relaxing and calming effect.

Makes 1–3 servings

$^{1}/_{2}$ **fennel bulb (approx. 3$^{1}/_{2}$ ounces) (use the rest in a roast vegetable combo to treat yourself)**

Wash, and remove the tough root bottom of the bulb and chop finely.

Steam for 5–7 minutes in an electric steamer until soft. (You can pan cook in enough boiling water to cover the fennel, but steaming will produce the best result.)

Purée, using the chopping attachment of a hand blender, until smooth, adding the stock collected in the steamer tray or pan to create a glossy finish.

Finally push through a fine sieve or finest-grade food mill disk.

Beet Purée

If you are fed up with all your baby food looking pretty much the same color then this is one to buck the trend. It's so colorful it comes with a diaper warning! Beets contain no fat but are a great source of fiber. Packed with iron and magnesium, beets are known as the vitality plant and have been used in the treatment of cancer, especially leukemia. If there was a food Oscars, this veg would definitely feel at home walking down the red carpet.

Like all root vegetables beets have a natural sweetness that your baby will love.

Makes 1–3 servings

1 large or 2 small fresh beets (approx. 3$^{1}/_{2}$ ounces)

Wash, top, tail, and peel the beets. Dice into $^{1}/_{8}$-inch cubes or use the coarse shredding attachment of a food processor.

In a small saucepan, bring just enough water to cover the beets to the boil. Add the beets, reduce to a gentle simmer,. and cook for 10–12 minutes until soft. (Although beets can be steamed, they tend to discolor the plastic of electric steamers, so stick with the pan method.)

Purée, using the chopping attachment of a hand blender, until smooth, adding the stock collected in the pan to create a glossy finish.

Finally push through a fine sieve or finest-grade food mill disk.

Diaper warning! Beets can give your baby red pee and poop. It's not dangerous, but can be a bit of a shock when you first see it.

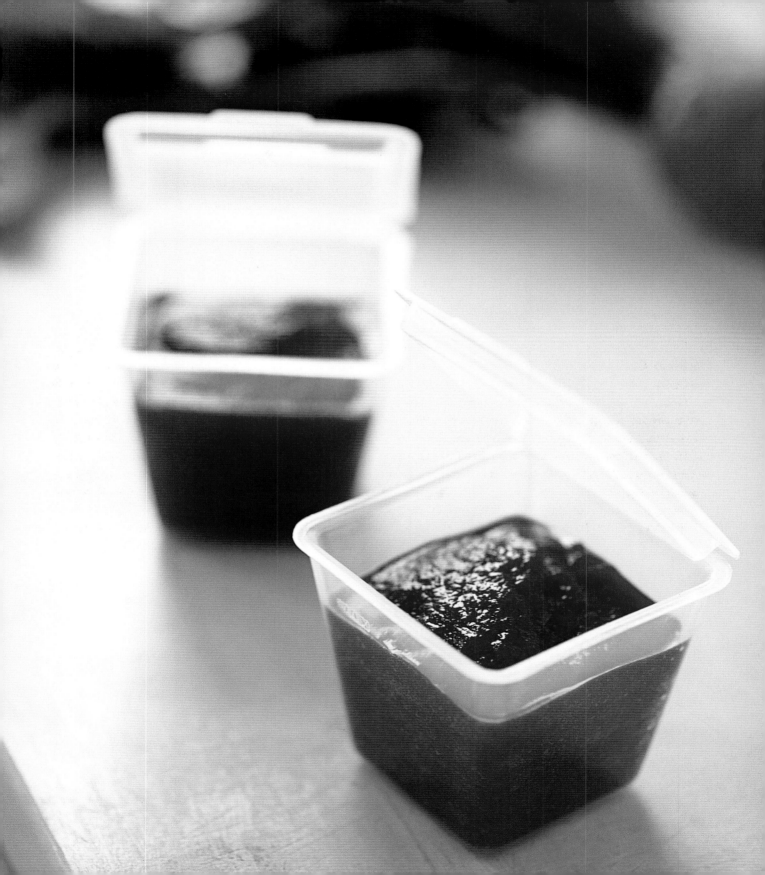

Spinach Purée

Spinach can have quite a strong taste, so choose baby rather than large leaf spinach because it's sweeter. I have kept the quantity very small as I find it's something of a "love-it or hate-it" purée. Try blending with baby rice, your baby's usual milk, or a tried-and-tested favorite purée to introduce for the first time.
Makes 1–2 servings

2 cups fresh baby spinach leaves

Thoroughly wash the leaves, removing any tough-looking stems and tearing any larger leaves in half.

For best results, steam for 5–7 minutes in an electric steamer. Alternatively, in a small saucepan, bring to the boil just enough water to cover, add the spinach, and simmer for 6–10 minutes until soft.

Purée, using the chopping attachment of a hand blender, until smooth, adding the stock collected in the steamer tray or pan to create a glossy finish.

Finally push through a fine strainer or finest-grade food mill disk to remove any stringy bits you may have missed.

Zucchini Purée

The zucchini is a summer squash. They are usually green or yellow and sold when they are about 5–6 inches in size. They're a good stage 1 weaning food since they don't have a strong taste and most babies will take to them with relish. If you are bored with orange-colored purées, this makes a bright green subtle-tasting purée.
Makes 1–3 servings

I small zucchini (approx. 3½ ounces)

If you can only find large zucchini, the skin may be a little tough—in which case, you'll need to peel. Otherwise simply wash, top and tail, then finely chop or grate.

Steam for 5–7 minutes in an electric steamer. Alternatively, in a small saucepan bring to the boil just enough water to cover, add the zucchini and simmer for 6–10 minutes until soft.

Purée, using the chopping attachment of a hand blender, until smooth, adding the stock collected in the steamer tray or pan to create a glossy finish.

Finally push through a fine strainer or finest-grade food mill disk.

String Bean Purée

These lean, mean fighting machines are bright, shiny, and glossy when fresh, but, like a prize fighter who has fought too many rounds, they start bulging and become leafy and limp when old. String beans are a good source of lutein, an antioxidant that is good for eye health.
Makes 1–3 servings

$1/3$ **cup fresh young string beans**

Wash and finely slice the beans, removing any tough stringy strands.

For best results, steam for 6–8 minutes in an electric steamer. Alternatively, in a small saucepan bring to the boil just enough water to cover, add the beans, and simmer for 8–10 minutes until soft.

Purée, using the chopping attachment of a hand blender, until smooth, adding the stock collected in the steamer tray or pan to create a glossy finish.

Finally push through a fine strainer or finest-grade food mill disk to remove any stringy bits you may have missed.

Potato Purée

I've met several parents who fully intended to make all their own baby food, only to start with potato and then vow never to purée again–either because they end up in a sticky mess or, very occasionally, because babies can be intolerant to them during the first weeks of weaning. I recommend that you hold off introducing potatoes until you and your baby are chugging away confidently with the other purées in this section.

Try potato on its own before introducing it as part of a stage 2 purée to check for any adverse reactions.

In its defense, the potato does contain the mood leveler vitamin B[3] (niacin) that helps to create the "happy" hormone serotonin. It is also a source of vitamin B, and is high in vitamin C as well as providing energy-rich carbohydrate.
Makes 1 serving

I small potato (approx. 2 ounces)

Wash the potato and peel unless you intend to bake it.

Pan cook the potato in just enough boiling water to cover. Or puncture holes in the potato with a fork and bake for 25 minutes at 300°F.

If baked, scoop out the soft flesh, then give it a brief purée in the chopping attachment of a hand blender. If you purée for too long, the starch is released and you'll end up with a goo resembling glue. Add a little boiled water if needed. If the cooked potato is very soft, you could omit the blending stage and simply push through a fine strainer or finest-grade food mill disk.

Fruit purées

If you are struggling with any of the veggie purées on the previous pages or you need to sweeten a later-stage meal the following fruit purées can be frozen and added as a natural sweetener. Just remember not to eat them all yourself.

Pear Purée

Pears are a soft, gentle first weaning food, with an extremely low likelihood of intolerance. Pears contain pectin, which helps those little bowels to start processing solids efficiently. Like most fruits, pears offer a rich source of vitamin C and iodine, which the thyroid gland craves to kick-start the metabolism and produce energy. Pears also contain small quantities of folic acid and iron.

Makes 1–3 servings

1 small ripe pear (approx. 3½ ounces)

Peel and carefully core the pear, making sure you have removed all the seed husks. Chop into very small chunks or grate directly into the boiling water.

To steam, follow the Apple Purée recipe (see right).

In a small saucepan, bring 1 tablespoon of water to a rolling boil. Add the pear and simmer for 8–10 minutes until the largest piece is soft.

Purée, using the chopping attachment of a hand blender, until smooth. Finally push through a fine strainer or finest-grade food mill disk.

Apple Purée

"An apple a day…" well, you know the rest. Once introduced to apples, most babies will love them in any shape or form throughout their lives. Like pears, apples contain pectin, a soluble fiber that helps to stimulate bacteria in the gut and improves food "elimination" (don't you just love the scientific word for poop). Apples also provide vitamin C and beta-carotene, a winning duo to bolster any fledgling immune system. I love using locally grown, seasonal apples—they remind me of my Grandma Daisy, who had a big tree that came into fruit to mark the beginning of fall. Look out for unusual varieties direct from the growers at your local farmers market—you'll be amazed how much the purées vary in taste, color, and texture.

Most commercial baby food companies use chemical treatments to prevent apples and pears from browning. This isn't necessary if the time between peeling and cooking is kept to an absolute minimum. By putting the prepared apple straight into boiling water, you'll find the purée stays pretty much the color nature intended.

Makes 1–3 servings

½ eating apple (3½ ounces)

Peel and carefully core the apple, making sure you have removed all the seed husks. Chop the apple into very small chunks or grate directly into the steamer compartment. Steam for 8–10 minutes.

For the saucepan method, follow the Pear recipe (see left).

Purée, using the chopping attachment of a hand blender, until smooth. Finally push through a fine sieve or finest-grade food mill disk.

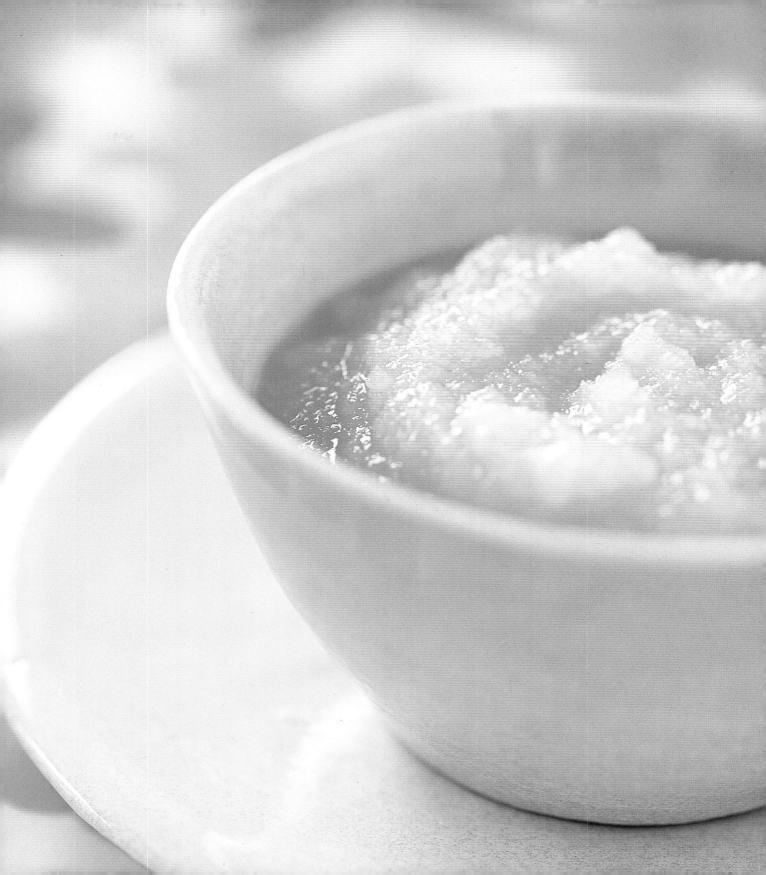

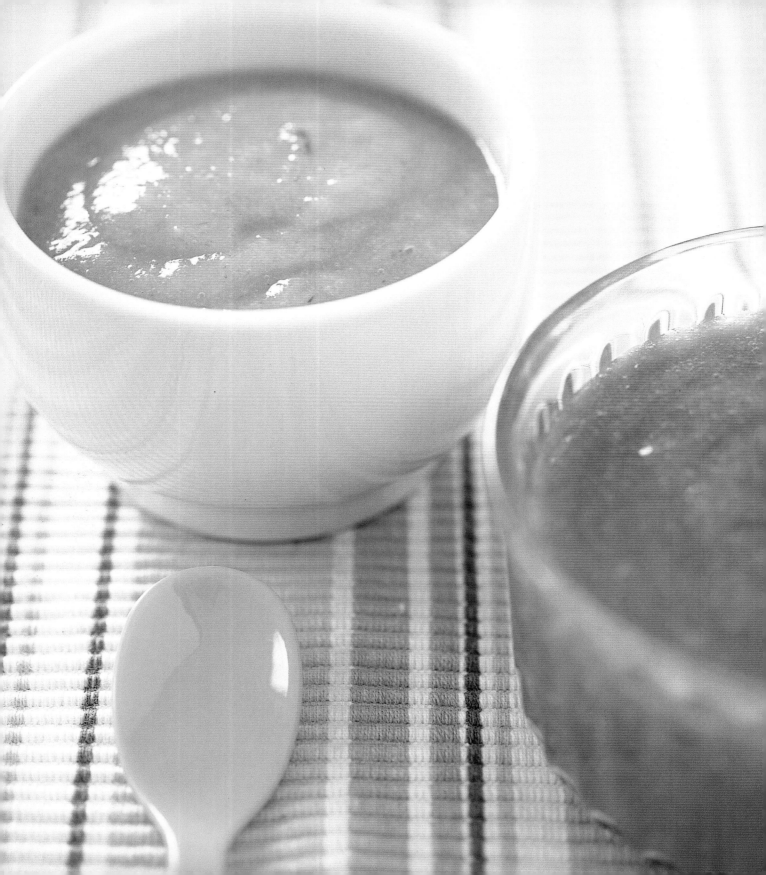

Nectarine or Peach Purée

These fruits are close sisters. Orange-colored varieties are full of, yet again, that immune award-winning team of beta-carotene and vitamin C, which will help your baby to ward off illnesses, particularly those who are being weaned off the immunological benefits of breastfeeding moms. When fully ripe, the flesh of these fruits is deliciously sweet, which your baby will adore. Surprisingly, they are also full of iron.

Makes 1–3 servings

½ **ripe peach (3½ ounces)**

Removing the skins of peaches (and plums) can be a messy business, resulting in lots of lost fruit, so try this way instead.

Run a sharp knife across the bottom of the fruit, place them in boiling water for about 30 seconds, remove carefully, and then dip them into iced water. Pour off the water and the skins should peel off easily.

Remove the pits and slice the fruit into a small saucepan, catching any juice as you go. Simmer, only adding a little water if necessary, until soft.

Purée, using the chopping attachment of a hand blender, until smooth. Finally push through a fine strainer or finest-grade food mill disk.

Plum Purée

Makes 1–3 servings

3–4 **ripe, naturally sweet plums**

Some plums have very thin skins, others are quite tough. If you can start to peel the skin (rather than it being so thin it immediately tears), follow the technique for removing the skins of peaches (see left), but plunge into very hot water rather than a rolling boil otherwise you'll end up with a squishy mess!

Remove the pits and slice the fruit into a small saucepan, catching any juice as you go. Simmer until soft.

Purée, using the chopping attachment of a hand blender, until smooth. Finally push through a fine strainer or finest-grade food mill disk.

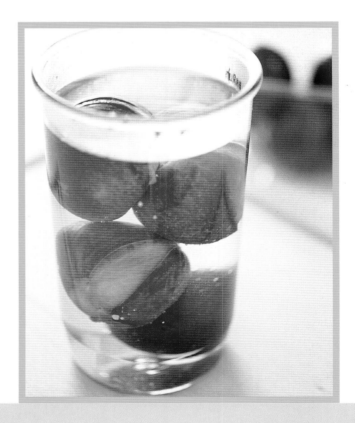

Mango Purée

Mangoes are one of life's treats. A juicy ripe mango not only gives your baby the immunological benefits of vitamin C and beta-carotene, but also calcium and magnesium, which are good for building strong bones and teeth. If your baby is having tummy trouble, mangoes may help, as they are highly alkaline and can balance any belly acidity issues.

I recommend cooking mango for the first few times—after that, as long as the mango is very ripe you can use the method for Papaya Purée on page 76.

If you're new to the world of mango, here's a crash course in how to tackle one. If it's ripe, the skin will give slightly when you gently push on it; it will also smell fragrant. Look out for a label on the fruit saying smooth or fibrous. If you get a choice, go for smooth. There is nothing wrong with the fibrous varieties, but, as the name suggests, they can leave tiny fibers in the purée that are perfectly safe but may be a bit of a surprise.

Makes 1–3 servings

3¹/₂ ounces ripe mango–use the rest of the fruit as a healthy and delicious treat for yourself

Mangoes have a large flat seed through the middle. Aim to cut either side of the seed, then score the flesh with a sharp knife. You should then be able to turn the skin back in on itself, so you can slice off the ready diced fruit (see photograph on page 95).

Chop the fruit up a little more over a small saucepan to catch the juice and simmer for 5 minutes until soft.

Purée, using the chopping attachment of a hand blender, until smooth. Finally push through a fine strainer or finest-grade food mill disk.

Dried Apricot or Prune Purées

Dried fruit condenses the goodness of the original fruit. Dried prunes (formerly plums) and dried apricots are an excellent source of iron, a.k.a. brain fodder. These fruits are rich in the dynamic, health-promoting duo vitamin C and beta-carotene. And, if that's not enough, they also have oodles of powerful potassium. Their natural sweetness makes them ideal for first purées. When choosing dried apricots, make sure that they're organic and are not sulphured. (Look out for those treated with sulphur dioxide as these can trigger latent asthma or allergies. Sulphur dioxide is used to keep the color bright orange, so choose dark brown dried apricots.) Prunes are a well-known laxative, so add small quantities of these purées to other fruit purées or use with baby rice and milk to begin with and assess the diaper damage.

Makes 1–3 servings

5–6 dried apricots or prunes (approx. 3¹/₂ ounces)

Wash and finely chop the fruit, checking for any bits of pit.

Bring 2–3 tablespoons of water to a full boil, then simmer the fruit for about 10 minutes until soft.

Purée, using the chopping attachment of a hand blender, then push through the finest-grade food mill disk, together with a little of the cooking water to make a smooth purée.

No-cook fruit purées

The following are no-cook purées. I do not recommend you start to wean your baby with these raw purées as cooked food is easier to digest. If you started weaning before 6 months I suggest that you wait until you are 4 weeks into weaning before you introduce these. Having said that, they are very easy to prepare and often adored by babies.

Banana Purée

Banana purée will probably be among your baby's—and child's—all-time favorite foods. From your point of view, bananas are perfectly portable, easy to turn into purée, and they come in their own sustainable, eco-friendly packaging. They are a rich source of complex carbs (the slow-releasing type), so give your baby a sustained slow release of sugar. Like other white-colored foods, they're a good source of potassium, which is good for nerve and muscle development. I am often asked if you can overdo the banana purée. According to oriental nutrition, bananas are described as "damp" and can cause babies (and adults) to produce too much mucus. In other words if your baby seems rather snotty, it might be worth turning down the volume of banana purée to see if it's the culprit.

Makes 1 serving (banana purée does not freeze well—but it's really easy to make fresh each time)

½ **small banana (approx. 2 ounces)**

Peel the banana, then blend until smooth using the chopping attachment of a hand blender. You will need to check for lumps before feeding the purée to your baby since you cannot strainer banana purée (if you try to push banana through a strainer, you'll end up with the most bizarre mix of gray liquid and revolting lumps—great!).

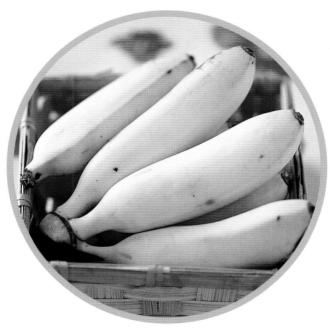

Avocado Purée

Is it a fruit? Is it a vegetable? No, it's an avocado. Whatever it is, remember the avocado has incredible powers. While rich in calories, an avocado is also one of the best sources of vitamin E, which helps with wound healing, a good complexion, and a robust immune system. Avocados also contain folic acid, which your baby needs as their iron sources reduce as they get older. If that wasn't enough, avocados are also full of monounsaturated fat, a good fat to give your baby energy. Oh—and they have the highest protein content of any fruit.

Makes 1 serving (avocado purée does not freeze well—but it's as easy to make fresh and you can treat yourself to some of the remaining fruit in a salad)

$1/4$–$1/2$ **avocado (leave the pit in the remaining fruit to reduce browning)**

Score criss-crosses through the flesh and use a spoon to scoop out the ready chopped pieces. Purée in the chopping attachment of a hand blender until smooth. Serve immediately since it will brown.

Papaya (Paw Paw) Purée

The papaya can grow from a seed to a 20-foot fruit-producing tree in less than 18 months. The fruits are usually sold when they are about the size of a pear and have an orangey skin. Don't be too disappointed when you cut into the flesh—the fruit contains quite a few black seeds which will need to be scraped away. The flesh should be a similar color to the skin and is a rich source of vitamins A and B.

Makes 1 serving

$1/4$–$1/2$ **papaya**

Remove the black seeds. Scoop out the flesh with a spoon and simply blend to a smooth purée using the chopper attachment of a hand blender.

Melon Purée

This is a delicious no-cook purée, so introduce it into your baby's diet once they're comfortable with cooked stage 1 purées and are chomping at the bit for some variety. Honeydews, watermelons, or cantaloupe, they're all great for puréeing. On purchase a melon should be fragrant and firm, and a little softness is a sign it is ripe. Always keep in the fridge because they go off quickly at room temperature, but before serving leave at room temperature for 1 hour to bring out the flavor. Melons are a rich source of vitamins A, C, and potassium but not good for freezing since they have a high water count.

Makes 1 serving (not suitable for freezing)

$1/8$ **medium melon**

Remove any seeds. Cut the flesh from the skin and simply blend to a smooth purée using the chopper attachment of a hand blender.

First spoonfuls

Choose the late morning/early lunch feed to introduce new foods when you and your baby feel more ready for new experiences. The volume of breast or formula milk needed depends on age and weight, so vary accordingly.

	Wake-up/ Breakfast	Late morning/Lunch	Mid-afternoon	Dinner	Bedtime
Days 1–2	Breast milk or formula milk (about 1 cup)	Breast milk or formula milk (about 1 cup) 1–2 teaspoons baby rice made with baby's usual milk	Breast milk or formula milk (about cup)	Breast milk or formula milk (about 1 cup)	Breast milk or formula milk (about ¾ cup)

First tastes

Introduce a purée over two consecutive days. If your baby prefers, mix the purée with a little baby rice.

	Wake-up/ Breakfast	Late morning/Lunch	Mid-afternoon	Dinner	Bedtime
Days 3–8	Breast milk or formula milk (about 1 cup)	Breast milk or formula milk (about 1 cup) 1–2 teaspoons of: Days 3 & 4 **Sweet Potato Purée** (p.60) Days 5 & 6 **Carrot Purée** (p.60) Days 7 & 8 **Pear or Apple Purée** (p.70)	Breast milk or formula milk (about ¾ cup)	Breast milk or formula milk (about 1 cup)	Breast milk or formula milk (about ½ cup)

Developing tastes

Remember all babies differ in preferences and appetites, so vary the purées and quantities to suit your baby. Follow this meal planner until you and your baby are comfortable with it, then move on to stage 2. Do not begin stage 2 until your baby is 6 months old. If your baby was an early weaner, repeat stage 1 until your child reaches 6 months.

	Wake-up/ Breakfast	Late morning/ Lunch	Mid-afternoon	Dinner	Bedtime
Weeks 2–4	Breast milk or formula milk (about 1 cup) Stage 1 **fruit purées** (see pp.70–76)	Breast milk or formula milk (about 1 cup) Stage 1 **vegetable purées** (see pp.60–69)	Breast milk or formula milk (about ¾ cup)	Breast milk or formula milk (about 1 cup) Optional: baby rice with your baby's favorite purée	Breast milk or formula milk (about ½ cup)

Exclusive breastfeeding is recommended for the first 6 months.
Drinking water should be boiled and cooled before giving to babies under 6 months.

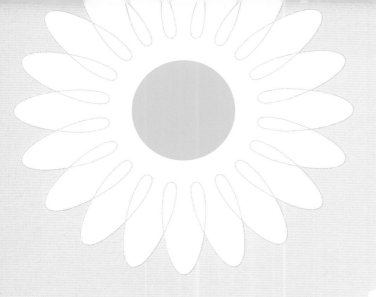

Stage two:
Textures and new tastes

Your child has become an eating machine and their first teeth are beginning to show. This section introduces new tastes and textures into their diet.

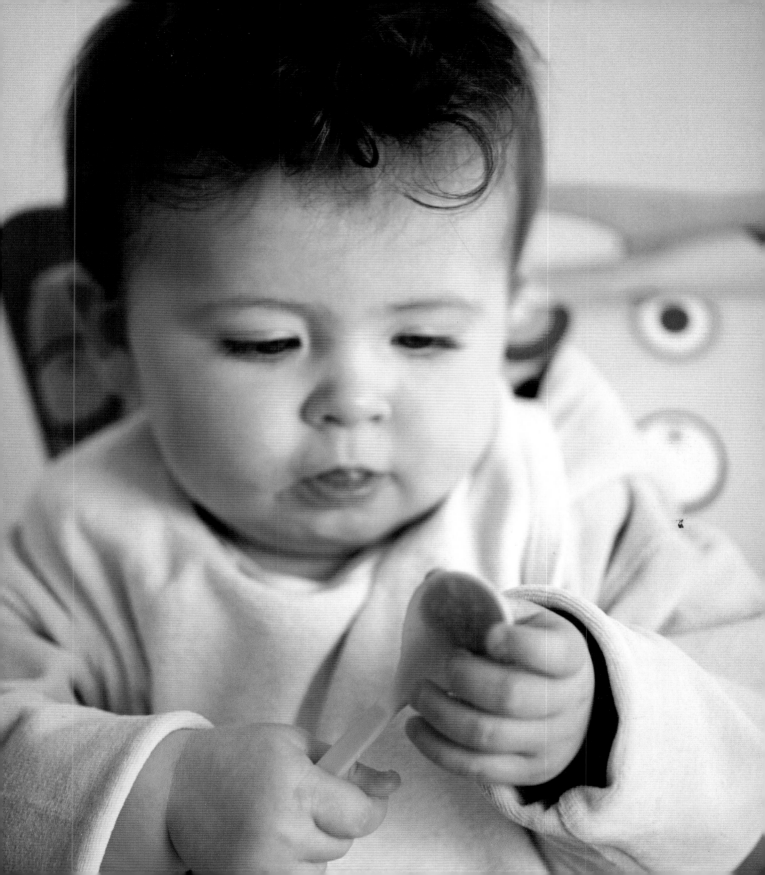

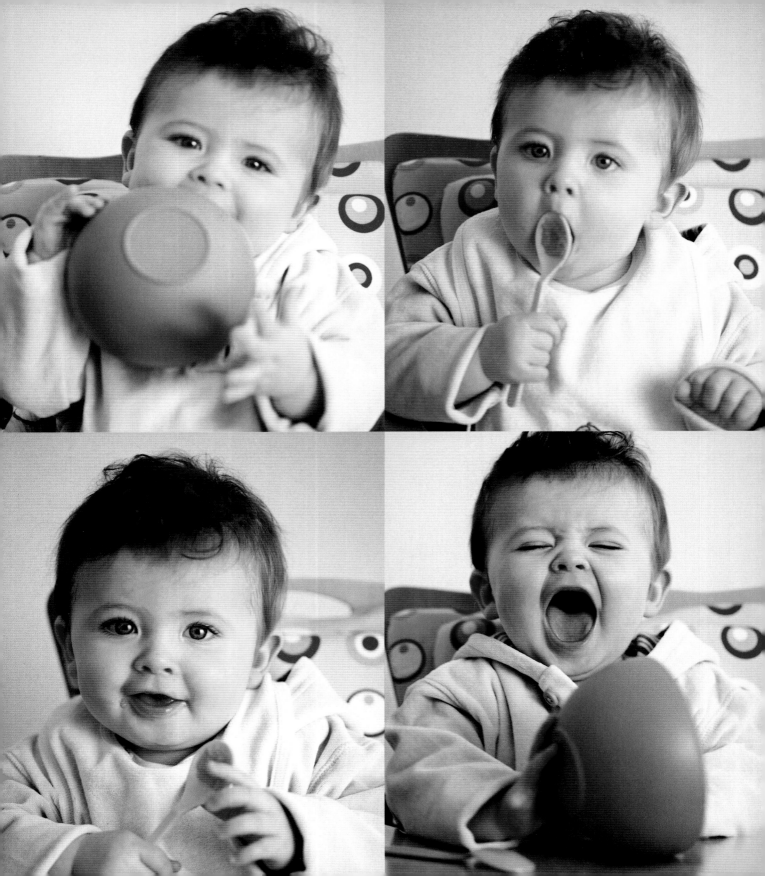

The second stage

Your baby's mouth has become a magnet—everything goes straight from their hand to their mouth. It's all part of their oral investigation of the expanding horizon around them. Your baby's muscular and skeletal development means that they now sit up confidently and are learning to reach, grasp, grab, pull, pinch, and hold. What's more, your baby's vision is also sharpening to an adult depth and they want to touch what they see. It's all exciting stuff and it means that it's high time to move on to the next stage of weaning, but do not begin this stage until your baby is 6 months old.

You'll both be feeling pretty comfortable with stage 1 purées, so it's time to get that little inquisitive mouth working harder. Learning to take "bits" into the mouth and knowing how to swallow them is a new skill that requires your baby to start finetuning some tongue control—as well as learning to eat, this stage is also thought to be an important step in learning to speak.

What to expect

Expect your stage 2 weaner to look at you with a confused face and then spit out the new textured purées. Don't be alarmed; although some babies take to texture like a duck to water, many are skeptical—it just requires more patience than easy-to-swallow, smooth purées. Choose the early feeds to introduce new textures as you did for new tastes—both you and your baby will feel fresher for a lesson in texture. Try not to feel pressured and if your baby is reluctant, go back to smooth purées for a day or two before trying again. It is an important step forward and worth persisting with.

First textures

Texture doesn't mean lumps. The purées should contain bits no bigger than $1/8$ inch, be soft enough to be squashed between your tongue and the roof of your mouth, and be swallowed without chewing. It's almost like "drinking" the purée in two swallows—the first for the wetter part of the purée, the second to finish off the squashy bits. Taste it yourself first: if you have to chew, the lumps are too big. Also, during stage 2 you will begin to recognize the recipes as the kind of food you would eat, admittedly through a straw, but it's a start.

Your trainee muncher is well on the way to solids, so confirm their new status in life by placing them at the top of the culinary world in a high chair.

Milk

Remember breast or formula milk is still your baby's primary food source and around $2^1/4$ cups should be consumed every day, including the milk used in cooking. Fresh cow's milk is a no-no for the first 12 months—which can cause some confusion as dairy products are often promoted as suitable for babies less than 1 year old. This is because the method used to make yogurts, fromage frais, hard cheeses, and the like makes them easier to digest, therefore safer for your baby than cow's milk. However, it is during stage 3 that these products really start to feature.

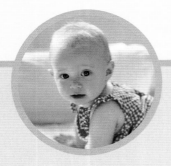

What's new in stage 2

Texture: purées, with bits in

Cereals: including oat-based oatmeal, millet and quinoa grain

Iron-rich foods become essential

Protein-rich foods: including lentils, tofu, poultry, meat, and fish

Eggs, but make sure they are well cooked (avoid if there is a family history of allergies)

Iron man

Their fledgling teeth and growing bones will need a significant nutrient boost to help sustain their development, so having the full complement of vitamins and minerals, iron, and proteins increases in importance.

In particular this stage sees the rising importance of iron and the introduction of proteins. Having been on solid foods for a month, your baby is now more active and going through an incredible rate of growth. You will have to increase the number of feeds and the amount they are eating. Your baby is born with iron reserves which in conjunction with breast milk or formula are sufficient up to 6 months. After that time iron is also needed from the diet.

Getting enough iron into your baby's system enables blood to carry oxygen around the body, feeding brain development. A lack of iron can mean that your child lacks

energy and, in the worst-case scenario, may develop anemia. This stage therefore sees plenty of iron-rich fruits and vegetables (apricots, peaches, raisins, prunes, bananas, avocados, spinach, and broccoli) and also marks the introduction of poultry and fish. Toward the end of stage 2 there is a recipe for your baby's first encounter with egg— the yolk is another iron-rich food.

It's also worth noting that vitamin C helps the absorption of iron so meals combining vitamin C and iron-rich ingredients are a winner, as is a serving of fruit purée as a dessert after an iron-rich main.

Vegetarian babies and iron

Parents wanting to bring up their child on a vegetarian diet should be aware there are two types of iron: non-heme and heme. Non-heme iron, found in vegetables, fruits, lentils, dried beans, and grain, is less readily absorbed by the body than the heme iron in rich animal products, so in order to make sure that your baby gets the necessary levels seek meal-planning advice from vegetarian organizations.

Protein pack

It's also time to introduce proteins, one of the body's essential building blocks. Start with simple fruit and vegetable sources such as lentil, quinoa, or tofu. Once your baby is doing well with these, you can then introduce recipes with good-quality organic chicken and fish.

You can substitute chicken for organic lean ground beef or lamb—both are rich in iron and protein— but avoid pork, including ham and bacon, because it's too high in salt and saturated fat.

Organic fish

Buying organic salmon and trout should be pretty easy, but finding organic white fish will prove difficult. To be certified organic, fish has to be farmed to make sure it is fed a purely organic diet—instead look for high-quality wild, white fish from sustainable stocks.

Teething

Ouch! Just as your baby is settling to a good night's sleep they start the painful business of teething. If you've ever had a toothache, you'll know how it hurts, so don't be surprised to find them stuffing anything into their mouths to alleviate the pain. Your baby may become irritable and eat erratically. Pressing hard, cool objects against their swollen gums helps them to cut their teeth. Their pearly white teeth should start popping up from 6 months onwards, and about 4 to 8 teeth are usually smiling at you by the age of 12 months.

The enamel on these newly erupting teeth is immature and vulnerable. They need careful looking after because they act as "holders" and guide in the adult teeth. Looking after your baby's teeth—and creating good food habits—can save a lifetime of dental work.

Tooth decay

Decay is caused by an acid in dental plaque, produced by bacteria feeding on the sugars we eat or drink. The acid attacks the hard enamel, producing holes and breaking down the softer dentine. One of the most common ways for teeth to be exposed to danger is from a baby's bottle.

Obvious drinks to watch out for are milk, formula, and fruit juice. The sugars in these liquids sit on infants' teeth and gums, feeding the bacteria that cause plaque.

Never allow your child to fall asleep with a bottle in their mouth. Tooth decay is also associated with children whose pacifiers are frequently dipped in honey, sugar, or syrup. The sweet fluids left in the mouth increase the chances of cavities developing while the infant is sleeping. Be careful also not to give your baby a sweet drink just before nap time since saliva production slows down during sleep, allowing the sugars to have their very own mouth party.

The more sugar your baby eats, the more likely it is that their teeth will suffer damage. Eating other foods at the same time as sugar or sugary foods dilutes the acid generated and reduces the harmful effects of sugar, so keep sugary foods for mealtimes.

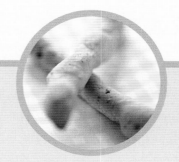

Teething-friendly foods

Freshly grated fruits or soft mushy fruits like mango or banana

Textured purées

For babies who are confident with finger foods, try:

Steamed carrot batons or vegetable sticks with a dip

Chilled cucumber, carrot, or fruit sticks

Thin breadsticks, rice cakes, or low-sugar rusks

Make sure you brush your baby's teeth thoroughly twice a day. Use a baby toothbrush with soft fibers or in times of very painful teething a clean, soft cloth wrapped around your finger. Just use a pea-sized blob of toothpaste. Interestingly, it's the use of fluoride as much as brushing that helps to prevent decay. Brushing last thing at night is very important, and you should do it for your child until they are 6 or 7 as most small people don't have the manual dexterity to brush properly. Studies show that children who brush more than once a day show the least decay.

If you want to minimize the amount of sugar in your baby's diet, remember that milk is high in lactose, so try dropping the night feeds. At night, the mouth produces less saliva than usual, which means that a sugary coating will cling to the teeth. If your baby insists on drinking at night, try a bottle of cooled boiled water instead.

Breakfast ideas

The works and a cup of coffee? Not quite at this age but the principle is the same. Walk past any diner at 7 in the morning and it'll be crammed with burly fellows in overalls readying themselves for a busy day of standing around, looking at problems, and saying, "This isn't going to be cheap!" The point is that a good, healthy feed in the morning will set your child up for the day and hopefully get them into a healthy routine for the rest of their life.

Banana and Prune Purée

Makes 1 serving (not suitable for freezing)

¹/₂ **cup prunes (or dried apricots, not treated with sulphur)**

¹/₂ **banana**

Cut the prunes into very small pieces. Bring to a boil just enough water to cover, add the prunes, and simmer until soft.

Purée with a hand blender together with the banana and serve as is, with baby's usual milk or, for the older child, swirled through natural yogurt.

Millet and Fruits

Makes 1 serving

¹/₂ **cup seasonal fruit or 2–3 frozen cubes of fruit purée**

2 **tablespoons millet flakes**

Wash, peel, and chop the fruit (this recipe works very well with apples, peaches, and even dried fruits).

In a saucepan, add enough water to cover the fruit, bring to a boil, add the fruit, and simmer until soft. Alternatively, defrost the cubes.

Sprinkle in the millet flakes, stirring continuously as it will thicken quickly. Add some of your baby's usual milk if the mixture becomes too thick.

Beginner's Oatmeal

Oats are not gluten free, although are thought to have a different type of gluten from wheat, and are therefore not supposed to cause the same digestive problems in gluten intolerant babies.

Makes 1 serving (not suitable for freezing if using banana)

¹/₂ **cup of your baby's usual milk**

¹/₄ **cup rolled oats**

2–4 **frozen cubes of your baby's favorite fruit purée or ¹/₂ small banana, mashed**

Heat the baby's milk in a saucepan, stirring in the oats. Bring to a boil then reduce to a simmer, stirring occasionally until it thickens, then melt in the fruit cubes or add the mashed banana.

Purée briefly with a hand blender if the texture is still a little too coarse for the weaning stage.

Allow to cool and serve.

No-gluten Muesli

Most breakfast cereals are wheat based and therefore high in gluten, and recently there has been a trend toward reducing or even excluding gluten in the first year. This recipe uses a couple of unusual grains that are gluten free as well as nutritionally packed with goodness. Quinoa is particularly useful since it provides essential amino acids normally only found in meat and dairy, as well as iron and calcium (so is particularly worth noting for parents bringing up their babies on a vegetarian diet). The added fruit helps the absorption of the minerals and brings vitamins C and D along to the breakfast party, making it a great way to start the day for grown-ups as well as babies.

Makes 1–3 servings

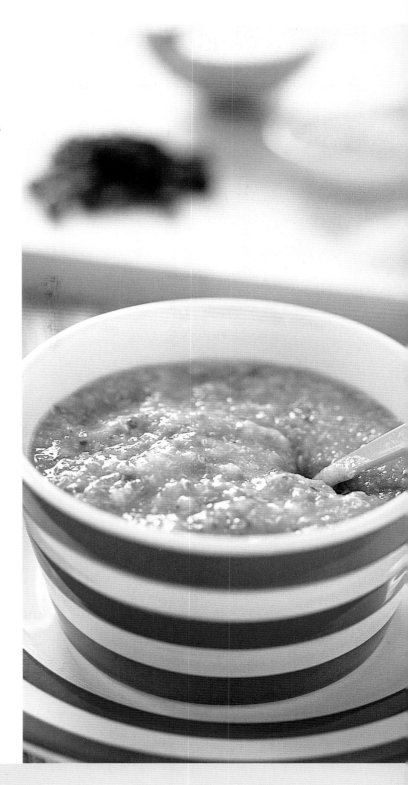

¼ cup quinoa grain

4 dried apricots (check they are not treated with sulfur) or ⅓ cup golden raisins

½ apple

1½ tablespoons millet flakes

Pinch of cinnamon (optional)

Cover the quinoa with water, bring to a boil, then simmer for 10 minutes.

Chop the apricots, then peel the apple and chop. Add the apricots and apple to the quinoa and simmer for a further 10 minutes until the grains are soft (they will become transparent). Add more water as needed. Stir in the millet flakes and cinnamon, if using, and gently cook for a further 3–5 minutes.

Use a hand blender to break down the grains, adding more boiling water to give the purée a glossy shine.

Serve on its own, mix in your baby's usual milk or mashed banana, or, for the older child, swirl with yogurt.

Freeze the remainder, but note that a little more water or your baby's usual milk may be needed after defrosting.

Vegetable and fruit combos

Your baby should be chomping at the bit by now, so it's time to up the ante on the texture. They will be comfortable with various individual fruits and vegetables in stage 1, so similarly at this stage if there is a new fruit or vegetable on the menu, combine it with other ingredients you know they like and introduce it into their diet at lunchtime so you can monitor any reactions. You can also start introducing a range of flavors in slightly more complicated recipes.

I suggest starting with Apple and Pear (see page 96) and Carrot and Sweet Potato (see below) since they are usually a safe bet for a child because the taste is quite sweet.

Carrot and Sweet Potato Purée

Sweet potatoes are easier to digest than standard potatoes and like carrots have a natural sweetness making both great stage 1 purées. This combo is our number one savory tip for introducing first textures—it's almost a stage 1.

The aim is to introduce texture gradually to get your baby used to dealing with bits.
Makes 1–3 servings

½ cup carrot	Chopped fresh cilantro to add
½ cup sweet potato	taste for the more confident
	weaner (optional)

Wash, then peel the carrots and sweet potato. Finely dice in a food processor or chop into approx ⅛ inch cubes.

Steam for 10–15 minutes or until the sweet potato is completely soft. The carrot should hold its shape but be easily squashed between your fingers or by your tongue on the roof of your mouth. Alternatively bring to a boil just enough water to cover the vegetables, add the vegetables, and simmer for 15 minutes. For the more confident weaner, add the cilantro for the last 5 minutes of cooking.

Purée with a hand blender or push through a strainer or food mill, adding the collected stock from the steamer tray or the water used to boil the vegetables to make a glossy purée.
Tip See page 39 for how to turn this into a delicious soup for adults.

Seasonal Root Vegetable Purée

Turnips, rutabaga, and parsnips may not play a large part in your diet, but don't overlook them for your baby. Take a taste yourself and you may be pleasantly surprised, because root vegetables are naturally sweet. However, they are particularly susceptible to pesticides, so search out organic, seasonal, locally grown treats whenever you can.
Makes 1–2 servings

⅓ cup carrot or parsnip	½ cup rutabaga or turnip or
½ cup sweet potato or	beets*
potato	

Wash and peel the vegetables (removing the tough/stringy cores if needed).

Finely chop in a food processor to make ⅛ inch dice or use a cheese grater to make fine strips. Steam for 10 minutes, or bring to a boil just enough water to cover the vegetables, add the vegetables, and cook until soft enough to squeeze between your fingers.

Purée with a hand blender or push through a strainer or food mill (if hand blending, potato will go sticky and gluelike if you overblend—stick to short blasts and stir to check for lumps).

*****Diaper warning!** See the beets warning on page 66.

Potato, Parsnip, and Pear Purée

This may seem an odd combination. Some people love it, others just can't get their heads round the taste. Whether it's a preconceived idea of fruit and vegetable not going together, I don't know, but just think of pineapples on baked ham and you start to understand where I'm heading with this. It's a nice one if your baby is struggling with vegetables since the parsnips have a natural sweetness and, combined with the potatoes, give a great texture. Don't blend it for too long as the starch will come out of the potatoes and you'll end up with a gluey mess. This recipe won a "Commended" at the Organic Food Awards in the UK.

Makes 1–3 servings

⅓ **cup potato**   ⅓ **cup ripe pear**
⅓ **cup parsnip**

Wash, peel, and chop the vegetables to ⅛ inch cubes—you may need to remove the hard core from the parsnip.

Next bring the potato to a rolling boil in just enough water to cover, then add the parsnips, and simmer both for about 6 minutes until they begin to soften.

Finally add the pear, return to a boil, and simmer for a further 4–5 minutes until all the cubes are soft.

If needed, purée with a hand blender or push through a strainer or food mill.

Broccoli, Cauliflower, and Potato Purée

This recipe always attracts a lot of questions, especially on how to cook the broccoli. Broccoli is a tricky one: Undercook and it can be too crunchy, overcook and it becomes waterlogged, loses its texture, goes grayish, and smells unpleasant. Cooked just right, however, broccoli has a fragrant aroma, a lovely texture, and is a lush green color. This is the real tester for a commercial baby food company—people who use processed baby food can't get over how our product actually smells of broccoli!

A waterlogged purée in this recipe usually means that the florets are too large and need to be cooked for too long to reach the required texture. The trick? Chop to a uniform ⅛ inch in a food processor, then cook in water already at a rolling boil or in a steamer at temperature.

Makes 1–3 servings

slightly more than ⅓ cup   ⅓ **cup broccoli**
   potato   ⅓ **cup cauliflower**

Wash and peel the potato. Rinse the broccoli and cauliflower, checking for any organic bugs.

Chop the potato, broccoli, and cauliflower using the grater blade of a food processor into ⅛ inch dice, or finely hand chop.

Tip the mixture into a pan containing 4–5 tablespoons of boiling water and cook for 8–10 minutes until the largest piece is soft. Or steam in an electric steamer.

If needed, purée with a hand blender or push through a strainer or food mill.

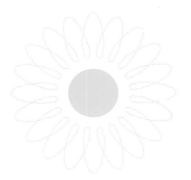

Pea and Bean Purée

Both vegetables are a great source of protein, fiber, and iron and since they have soft textures they make a wonderful purée. If fresh or frozen peas, rather than canned, are used, they have a wonderfully vibrant color and a really fresh taste.
Makes 1–3 servings

1/2 cup peas, snow peas or sugar snap peas (fresh or frozen)	1/3 cup string beans

Rinse the peas, top and tail the snow peas or sugar snaps, if using. Rinse, top, tail, and remove any tough, stringy bits from the beans.

   Steam or simmer for 8–10 minutes . Push through a food mill to remove any hard pea husks, adding a little of the steamer stock or cooking water to produce a glossy textured purée.

Sweet Red Pepper, Carrot, and Cauliflower Purée

This combo makes an impressively colorful purée—you can replace the red pepper with yellow, orange or even green peppers, but note green pepper is not as sweet.
Makes 1–2 servings

1/3 cup carrot	1/4 cup red pepper
1/3 cup cauliflower	

Wash, peel, and grate the carrot. For best results, steam the carrot while you prepare the cauliflower and red pepper.

   Wash the cauliflower and pepper, removing the seeds and the white pith. Finely hand chop or put through the coarsest grater attachment of a food processor.

   Add to the carrot and continue to steam for a further 6–8 minutes until the largest piece is tender. Blend to a purée.

Spinach and Sweet Potato Purée

Spinach has less ready-to-use iron than dried apricots and tuna but is brimming with calcium, magnesium, potassium, and folic acid. Its real strength is vitamin A, particularly lutein, which helps eyesight. Spinach has a slightly bitter taste, which is why I suggest using sweeter baby spinach and matching it with a vegetable that is naturally sweet.
Makes 1–2 servings

1/2 cup sweet potato	3/2 cup fresh baby spinach

Wash, peel, and grate or chop the sweet potato. Wash the spinach, checking over for any bugs.

   Although this can be cooked in a saucepan, steaming is better since the nutrients in spinach are easily destroyed by overcooking. For best results, steam the sweet potato for 5 minutes, then add the spinach leaves and cook together for 3–5 minutes, until the largest pieces of sweet potato can be squashed between your finger and thumb.

   Combine with a little of the steamer stock, using a hand blender.

Leek, Carrot, and Potato Mash

Makes 1–2 servings

1/3 cup carrot	1/4 cup leek
a little over 1/3 cup potato, (or sweet potato)	1 tablespoon baby's usual milk

Wash, peel, and finely chop (1/8 inch cubes) the carrot and potato. Bring 2 tablespoons of water to a boil, add the carrot and potato, and simmer for 5 minutes.

   Rinse the leek, cut lengthwise then crosswise into dice and add to the potato and carrot together with the milk. Simmer for a further 5 minutes until the largest piece is tender, then mash, adding more baby's milk as needed.

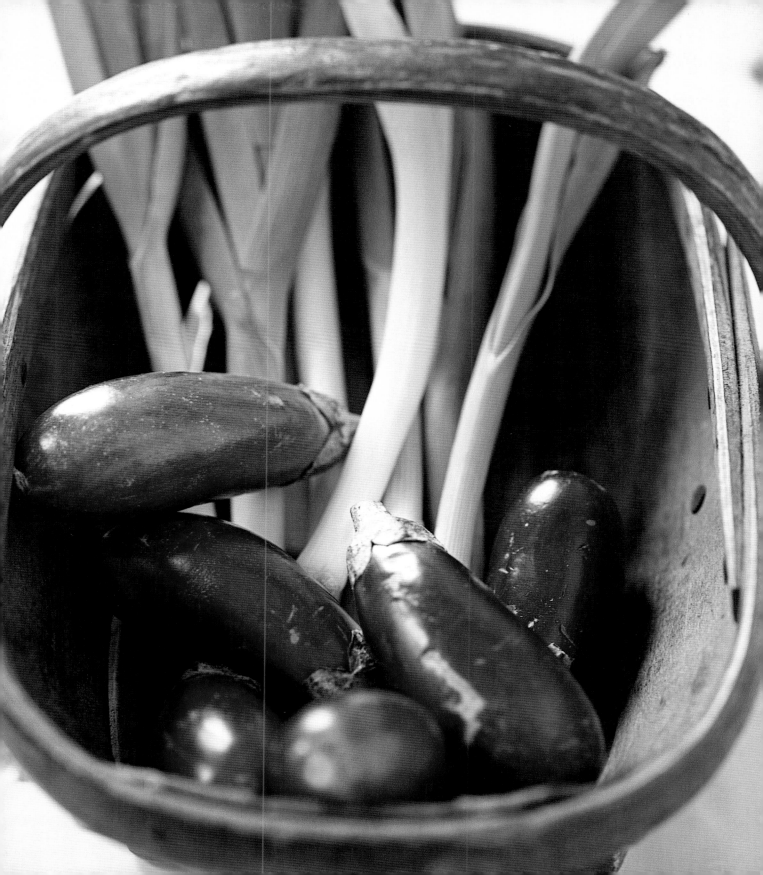

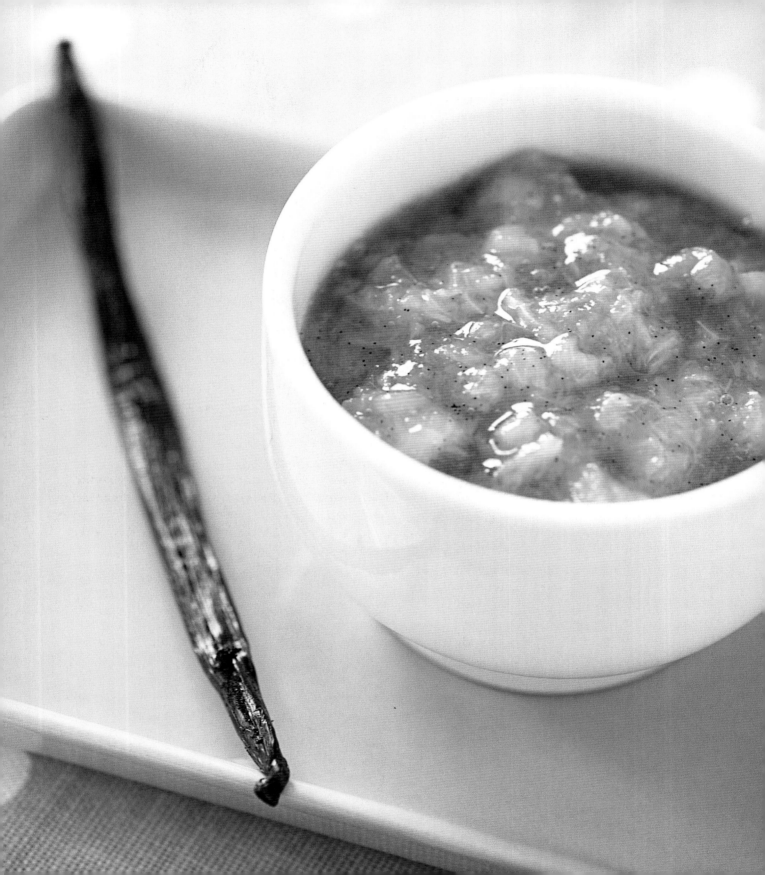

Peach, Plum, and Vanilla Purée

A real summer treat. The purée has a wonderfully rich color and a sweet and sour taste that will make your baby pucker up as the sharpness of the plums kicks in. Get the camera out! Their face will be a treat, but after the initial surprise, they'll be reaching out for the spoon to get more. The vanilla adds another dimension and this combination really gets all of the mouth's taste buds working. Older children and adults love this either drizzled over ice cream or on its own. This recipe picked up a "Highly Commended" at the U.K. Organic Food Awards.

Makes 2–3 servings

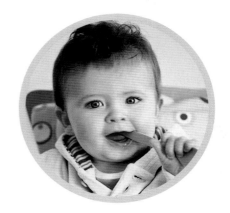

2 small or 1 large peach	1 vanilla pod, 1/2–1 inch
2–3 plums	length

Removing the skins of peaches and plums can be a messy business ending up with lots of lost fruit, so try running a sharp knife across the bottom of each fruit, place in water on a rolling boil for about 30 seconds, remove carefully, then dip them into ice water. Pour off the water and the skins should peel off easily.

Remove the pits and slice the fruit into a small saucepan, catching any juice as you go.

Split the vanilla pod, down the middle, on a chopping board. Bring the tip of the knife down the inside of the pod and the sticky black vanilla seeds will collect on the knife. Add to the peaches and plums.

Simmer, only adding a little water if necessary, until soft. Mix in a blender to a slightly textured purée. The slight flecking through the mixture is the vanilla.

Tip For a grown-up treat, pour the mixture into a plastic container and freeze for 30 minutes. Remove and fluff up with a fork, freeze again, and repeat until it forms a granita. Serve in a fancy glass topped with a sprig of mint.

Plum and Melon Purée

Makes 1 serving (not suitable for freezing, but is easy to make)

1/3 cup plum purée (see page 73) or 2–3 frozen cubes	1/3 cup melon (honeydew or galia)

Defrost the plum purée, if necessary, then pour into the chopping bowl attachment of a hand blender.

Remove any seeds from the melon, then scoop the melon flesh from the skin and add to the blender bowl. Blend for a few seconds to make a slightly textured purée.

This is also delicious made with fresh, ripe peaches or nectarines instead of plums.

Nectarine and Dried Apricot Purée

Iron-rich and delicious.
Makes 1 serving

3–4 dried apricots (pitted and not treated with sulfur)   1 ripe nectarine

Wash the apricots and chop, removing any bits of the pit or stem. Place in a small pan with 2 tablespoons of boiling water and simmer until soft and plump, about 7–9 minutes. If you are planning to make a large batch, I'd recommend washing then soaking the apricots overnight; as this softens the dried fruit and reduces the cooking time.

Wash and peel the nectarine if the skin is tough. Cut in half to remove the pit, slice the fruit, and add to the apricot. Continue to cook for a further 2–3 minutes.

Remove any larger bits of nectarine skin then combine using a hand blender.

Tip Treat yourself and any older kids to some of this purée swirled with yogurt or on ice cream.

Dried Fruit Compote

Dried fruit is handy to have in the cupboard, especially when time is not on your side. A good mix of prunes, dried apricots, currants, dried apple, golden raisins, and raisins will provide calcium, iron and vitamins A, B^2, and B^6.
Makes 1 serving

½ cup mixed dried fruit (currants, prunes, apple, golden raisins, and raisins, apricots—check they have not been treated with sulfur)

If you have the time or inclination soak the dried fruit mixture overnight to soften, then simply rinse and cover with ½ cup boiling water. Cover and allow to cool, then refrigerate overnight.

Or rinse, then chop the dried fruit mixture into ⅛ inch dice—you can do this by hand or in a food processor. Bring ½ cup water to a boil in a small saucepan. Add the dried fruit to the water and reduce to a simmer. Cover and simmer for about 20 minutes, adding a little more water as needed, until the largest piece is soft.

For added creaminess, add a couple of tablespoons of your baby's usual milk instead of the extra water.

If needed, mix using the blender.

Pear, Raisin, and Golden Raisin Purée

In the great tradition of the American dream, the raisin (although there are records of sun-dried grapes dating back to 1500 BC) has been written into American folklore by a supreme piece of opportunism. After a heatwave in San Francisco in 1873, the grapes left shrivelled and withered were relabeled by a grocer as a "Peruvian Delicacy" and flew off the shelf. **Makes 1 serving**

1 ripe pear
1 tablespoon raisins and
  golden raisins

Pinch of cinnamon (optional)

Wash and peel the pear. Cut in quarters, cut out the core, and finely chop.

Bring a couple of teaspoons of water to a boil, add the pear, and reduce to a simmer. If the pear is not particularly juicy, you will need to add a little extra water.

Halve or quarter the raisins and golden raisins and stir into the pear with the cinnamon, if using. Cover and simmer for 8–10 minutes.

Mix, using a hand blender before serving.

Strawberry and Banana Purée

If your child is hungry and making a racket, it's time to serve up that great Wimbledon institution: strawberries (without the cream and champagne). Your child will love these sweet little summer fruits (see below for other suggested fruits) which are rich in vitamin C and beta-carotene.

These innocent little fruits (and berries and kiwis) come with a warning because they can cause irritation in children with sensitive skin or eczema. Mixing them with banana is a good idea because you can blend in just a half or a quarter of a strawberry. Watch out for soreness around the mouth or blistering.
Makes 1 serving

1 small banana

½ cup strawberries or kiwi
  (or other berries, including
  blueberries, raspberries, or
  blackberries)

Simply blend the peeled banana with the washed berries until smooth or slightly textured.

If preparing for older children, simply mash together with a fork.

This recipe is a great dip for older children (see page 128) and also a fantastic substitute for sugary jams and spreads.

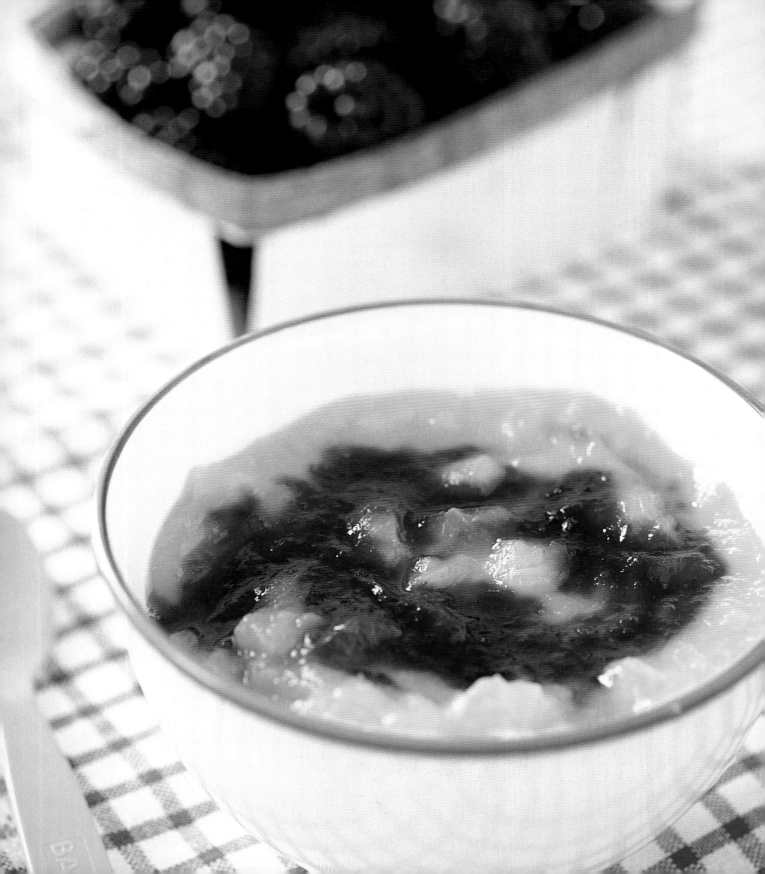

Mango with Blackberry Ripple

Part of learning to enjoy eating is the visual experience as well as the taste. These two purées have strong contrasting colors and make a feast for the eyes as well as the tummy.
Makes 1–3 servings

½ small ripe mango (if there is a choice select smooth rather than fibrous flesh)

½ cup fresh blackberries

Cut the mango in half lengthwise either side of the large pit. Score the inside of the flesh and turn the skin back on itself (see photograph below). Using a small sharp knife, slice the cubes off the skin. (If the mango is not ripe enough this may not work—in which case you'll have to peel and slice the fruit off the pit.)

Either steam the mango flesh or simmer in a little boiling water (as little as possible) until very soft. Purée in the chopping bowl of a hand blender, keeping a little texture.

Wash the blackberries and simmer in ½ tablespoon of water for 8 minutes. Push the fruit through a fine strainer with the back of a metal spoon or use the finest grade of a food mill to remove the seeds.

Drop a few spoonfuls into a serving of mango purée and swirl round with a spoon. This can be frozen as separate ice cubes, or half fill with the mango purée and cover with the blackberry purée to make two-tone blocks.

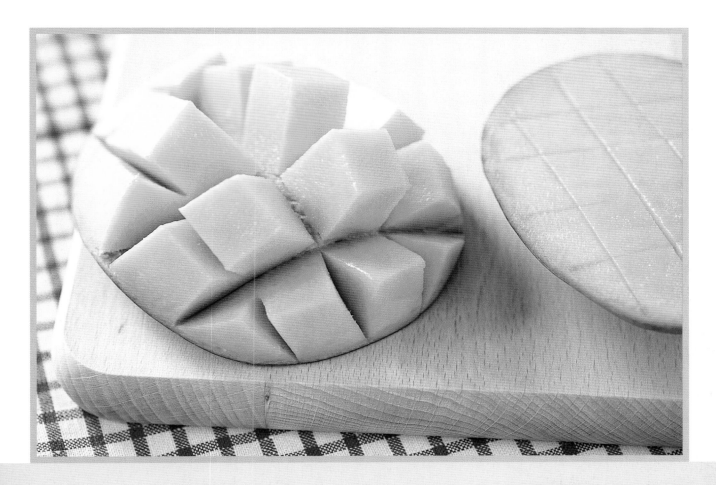

Apple and Mango Purée

This is simply delicious, and being honest there are times when I'll venture off to the freezer and defrost some to eat with vanilla ice cream. This is a great, easy weaner for your baby, with a natural sweetness they will love. Apples have a grainy texture while the mangoes are more stringy, but together they are a perfect combo for a child who is being launched into the world of texture. Mangoes are rich in vitamin C and beta-carotene and also contain calcium and magnesium which help to build strong bones and teeth. Mangoes are highly alkaline so will help balance out any acidity in your baby's stomach.

Makes 1 serving

1 small apple   **$\frac{1}{2}$ cup mango**

Core and peel the apple, making sure you remove all the seeds and husks.

Bring 1 tablespoon of water to a boil, then grate the apple into the boiling water—this will keep browning to a minimum.

Finely slice the mango into the apple—if the mango is very ripe, hold it over the pan so you capture all the juice. Or very briefly blend with a hand blender and pour the juicy mix into the pan. Simmer for 6–8 minutes until the apple is soft, then push through a food mill or give a short, sharp turn with the blender.

Apple and Pear Purée

Like the Carrot and Sweet Potato Purée, this is a simple combination of purées that you know your child is already comfortable with. I recommend having a stock of this in the freezer. It is great for filling a gap if your baby is screaming the house down.

Makes 1 serving

1 medium apple   **1 medium ripe pear**

If you have an apple corer, run it down the middle of the apple. Quarter the pear and remove the core. Make sure you remove all the seeds, pith, and the stem. Then peel the apple and pear and dice into $\frac{1}{8}$ inch squares.

Steam or pan cook with just a couple of teaspoons of boiling water for 10 minutes (you'll only need more if the pear is not very juicy), then push through a food mill or give a short sharp mix with a hand blender.

Avoid making the purée too smooth—this non-challenging purée is great for a first lesson in texture.

Weeks 4–6: First Textures

Timings and recipes are a rough guide, but this meal planner begins to shape into a more grown-up pattern of mealtimes. The volume of breast or formula milk needed depends on age and weight, so vary accordingly.

If your baby is struggling to cope with these textures, try puréeing a little more, or go back to very smooth for two days, then try again. Introduce new tastes and textures in the morning or at lunchtime.

Remember to include a drink of water with mealtimes.

	Wake-up	Breakfast	Lunch	Mid-afternoon	Dinner	Supper	Bedtime (optional)
Day 1	Breast milk or formula milk (1 cup)	Apple and Pear Purée (see p.96)	Carrot and Sweet Potato Purée (see p.86)	Breast milk or formula milk (3/4 cup)	Butternut Squash Purée (see p.64)	Breast milk or formula milk (3/4 cup)	Breast milk or formula milk (1/3 cup)*
Day 2	Breast milk or formula milk (1 cup)	Apple and Mango Purée (see p.96)	Seasonal Root Vegetable Purée (see p.86)	Breast milk or formula milk (3/4 cup)	Avocado Purée (see p.76)	Breast milk or formula milk (3/4 cup)	Breast milk or formula milk (1/3 cup)*
Day 3	Breast milk or formula milk (1 cup)	Apple and Pear Purée (see p.96)	Broccoli, Cauliflower, and Potato Purée (see p.87)	Breast milk or formula milk (3/4 cup)	Mashed Banana (see p.75)	Breast milk or formula milk (3/4 cup)	Breast milk or formula milk (1/3 cup)*
Day 4	Breast milk or formula milk (1 cup)	Nectarine and Dried Apricot Purée (see p.92)	Potato, Parsnip, and Pear Purée (see p.87)	Breast milk or formula milk (3/4 cup)	Carrot Purée (see p.60)	Breast milk or formula milk (3/4 cup)	Breast milk or formula milk (1/3 cup)*
Day 5	Breast milk or formula milk (1 cup)	Apple and Mango Purée (see p.96)	Squash and Red Lentil Purée (see p.99)	Breast milk or formula milk (3/4 cup)	Carrot and Sweet Potato Purée (see p.86)	Breast milk or formula milk (3/4 cup)	Breast milk or formula milk (1/3 cup)*
Day 6	Breast milk or formula milk (1 cup)	Pear, Raisin, and Golden Raisin Purée (see p.93)	Minty Pea and Potato Purée (see p.103)	Breast milk or formula milk (3/4 cup)	Seasonal Root Vegetable Purée (see p.86)	Breast milk or formula milk (3/4 cup)	Breast milk or formula milk (1/3 cup)*
Day 7	Breast milk or formula milk (1 cup)	No-gluten Muesli (see p.85)	Squash and Red Lentil Purée (see p.99)	Breast milk or formula milk (3/4 cup)	Mashed Banana (see p.75)	Breast milk or formula milk (3/4 cup)	Breast milk or formula milk (1/3 cup)*

* Optional, although many babies find it a comforting part of their bedtime routine

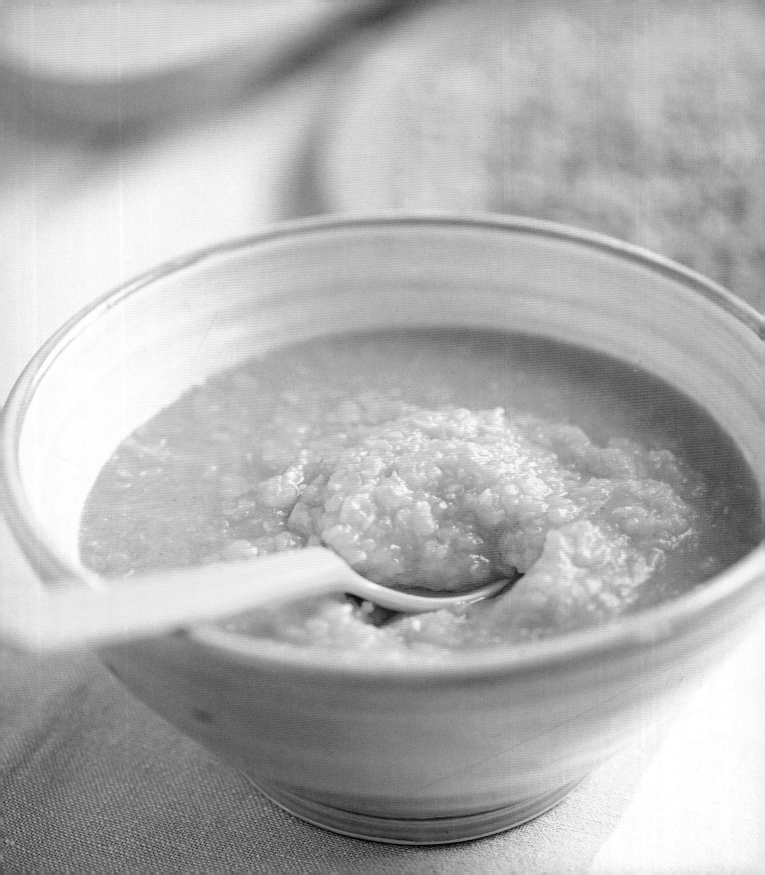

Introducing proteins

Our body needs 22 amino acids to run efficiently but only produces 13, so the way to get them is to introduce protein into the diet. Here are some great vegetable meals packed full of protein, followed by some fish and meat options.

Squash and Red Lentil Purée

You might expect one of the desserts to be my favorite, but this savory treat gets my lips smacking and stomach rumbling. With a homey, comforting aroma and heart-warming taste, it's won U.K. Organic Food Awards two years running including "Overall Winner of the Babyfood" category. Not only is this recipe simple to make, lentils introduce building block proteins into your baby's diet.
Makes 1–2 servings

¼ cup dried red lentils

½ cup squash (butternut squash is best)

Rinse the lentils in a strainer with cold water. In a clean saucepan add enough cold water to cover the lentils and bring gently to a boil. Add more water as needed. Cut the squash in half and scoop out the seeds. Lay the squash flat side down on a clean chopping board and remove the skin with a potato peeler. Either chop to a fine dice or use a food processor to produce ⅛ inch dice.

Add the squash to the lentils and bring to a rolling boil, then reduce to a simmer for a further 10 minutes, stirring occasionally, until the lentils and squash are soft enough to be squashed between your tongue and the roof of your mouth. The lentils will change from opaque to semi clear.

Push through a food mill or a metal strainer or quickly combine with a hand blender.

Tip Make up a large batch and use some for a comforting grown-up soup—simply add some stock (see page 118) and a little seasoning.

Dhal

Makes 1–2 servings

¼ cup dried red lentils

½ cup water

2 tablespoons onion or leek

½ teaspoon fresh parsley

Pinch of ground cumin

Pinch of ground cinnamon

Rinse the lentils thoroughly. In a saucepan, add enough water to cover the lentils and simmer for 15 minutes.

Finely chop the onion and parsley, and stir into the lentil mix with the cumin and cinnamon. Simmer for a further 10 minutes, adding more water as needed, until the lentils are soft enough to be squashed between your finger and thumb.

If the onion is chopped small enough and the mixture has been sufficiently cooked, further blending won't be needed; simply cool and serve or freeze.

Kiwi, Prune, and Tofu Purée

Furry brown kiwis are actually a berry, which is why kiwis are nutritionally different and superior to other fruits. Looks, you see, just like Clark Kent, are deceiving. By day the kiwi looks like a boring soul in a frumpy brown suit, but come dinner time, it's changed into a green superfood. Just one serving of kiwi fruit will give you 10 percent of your recommended daily allowance for vitamin E and your full day's vitamin C quota. A kiwi also contains more vitamin C than an orange and more potassium than a banana. The tiny black seeds are also a rich source of essential fatty acid which is rarely found outside seeds, oils, and nuts.

Note: some children are sensitive to kiwi fruit—introduce a small amount early in the day and monitor for any adverse reaction.

Makes 2–3 servings

¼ cup dried prunes, stoned   **2 tablespoons tofu**
1 kiwi fruit

Rinse the prunes, checking for any bits of pit or stem and chop in small pieces.

In a small pan, bring just enough water to cover the prunes to a boil, add the prunes and simmer for 10 minutes until soft and plump.

Peel the kiwi or cut in half and scoop out the flesh with a teaspoon and put into the chopping bowl of a hand blender. Add the tofu and the prunes, and blend, adding the water the prunes were cooked in as needed, until it is the right texture for your baby.

Tofu, Fennel, and Spinach Purée

Tofu is made from soybean curd, and is a good way to introduce protein into your baby's diet. Soybeans are soaked, crushed and heated to produce soy milk to which a coagulating agent, calcium sulphate or calcium chloride, is added. The soy curd is then pressed to give tofu. Tofu tends be fairly bland in taste and is best used in recipes where flavor is imparted by other ingredients. This is why it works well with fennel and spinach, both of which have strong flavors. At a later stage in your child's diet, firm tofu may be stir- or deep-fried, sautéed, or steamed and added to salads or casseroles. As well as having a high protein content, tofu also contains calcium, iron, and vitamins B^1, B^2 and B^3.

Makes 1–2 servings

½ fresh fennel bulb   **⅓ cup spinach leaves (preferably baby spinach as it is slightly sweeter)**
                                       ⅓ cup tofu

Wash and finely chop the fennel into approximately ⅛ inch cubes and steam for 5 minutes.

Wash the spinach leaves and add to the fennel. Steam for a further 5 minutes. Drain the tofu and roughly chop. Combine the steamed fennel and spinach with the tofu in the chopping bowl of a hand blender and mix, adding, if needed, a tablespoon of the collected stock from the steamer or boiled water.

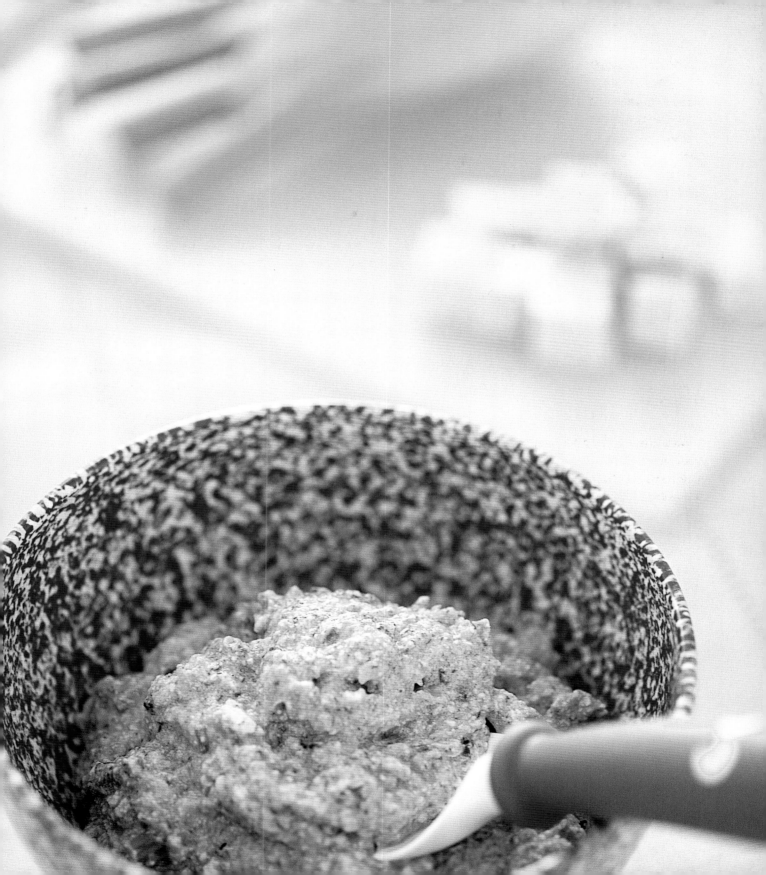

Simple Savory Quinoa Purée

Quinoa has very little flavor of its own so it works well in savory and sweet dishes. If this is the first time you are introducing tomato, as with other new foods, try a little at a midday meal so you can check for any intolerance. Also note the same care should be taken when introducing raw tomatoes for the first time; even if your baby is fine with cooked tomatoes, some babies (and adults) have an adverse reaction when tomatoes are eaten raw.

Makes 1 serving

1 tablespoon quinoa
¼ cup squash (butternut or
   red kuri)

2–3 cherry tomatoes
¼ cup zucchini

Cover the quinoa with water, bring to the boil then simmer for 10 minutes.

Peel the squash and chop into ⅛ inch dice, then add to the quinoa and simmer for a further 5 minutes until the grains and squash are soft (the quinoa will go transparent).

Purée the tomatoes and zucchini in the chopper attachment of a hand blender to form a coarse paste and pour into the pan. Cook for 5 minutes, stirring frequently. Add a little more water as needed.

Serve as is or give another quick buzz with the blender if your baby isn't ready for the bitty texture.

Quinoa, Rhubarb, and Vanilla Purée

Quinoa dates back to 2700 BC in China where it was cultivated for its purgative medicinal purposes, while rhubarb is native to the Incas of South America. Rhubarb is made up of 95 percent water but is a fair source of potassium, contains small amounts of vitamins and is low in sodium. Rhubarb is also rich in vitamin C, dietary fiber, and calcium. Rhubarb stalks can be a little tart so taste and select the sweetest bits. Only the stalks are edible, so don't use the leaves or roots.

Makes 1–2 servings

1 tablespoon quinoa
½ inch vanilla pod

½ cup rhubarb

Rinse the quinoa and split open the vanilla pod. Heat both ingredients in a pan with 2–3 tablespoons of water. Bring to a boil, cover, and reduce to a simmer for 5–10 minutes.

Slice the rhubarb thinly and stir into the mix. Simmer for 8–10 minutes until the grains are transparent and the rhubarb soft. Combine in the chopping bowl of a hand blender.

Tip If the rhubarb is particularly tart, stir in a couple of teaspoons of a sweeter purée such as pear, apple, or peach.

Minty Pea and Potato Purée

A refreshing combo: Peas contain protein but not all the essential amino acids. For more information, see page 17.
Makes 1–2 servings

½ cup potato
  or sweet potato
⅓ cup fresh or frozen peas

2–3 leaves of fresh mint (or
  pinch of dried)

Wash, peel, and finely chop or grate the potato. If using fresh peas, rinse with the mint leaves. Steam both ingredients for 10 minutes. Alternatively bring to a boil just enough water to cover the ingredients, add the ingredients, and simmer gently. When the largest piece of potato is soft, then blend to the right texture for your baby.

When serving, make sure all the whole peas have been mashed. If not, squash with the back of a spoon before giving to your baby.

Beet, Apple, and Butterbean Purée

Makes 1–2 servings

1 small beet*
½ medium apple

⅔ cup lima beans (canned, in
  water, or prepared as
  instructed on package)

Wash and peel the beet and chop into ⅛ inch dice, and heat in a pan with 2 tablespoons of boiling water.

Wash, core, and peel the apple then grate into the simmering beet. Simmer for a further 8 minutes.

Rinse the lima beans and add to the mixture and simmer for a further 2 minutes to heat through.

Give the mixture a quick buzz using the hand blender to make a slightly textured purée.

*Diaper warning! See page 66.

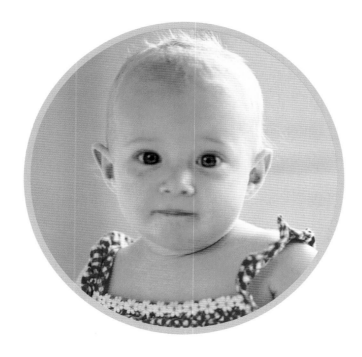

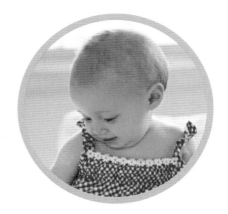

Chicken for Beginners

Makes 2–3 servings

¼ **pound chicken breast,**
  skinless

½ **red pepper**
¼ **avocado**

Wash and dice the chicken and red pepper into small cubes. Steam the chicken and pepper for 8–10 minutes, checking the chicken is cooked thoroughly.

Blend the chicken and pepper with 1–2 tablespoons of stock (from the steamer) or boiled water.

Divide the mixture into two and set aside half to freeze (avocado doesn't freeze very well, so it should be added just before serving).

Roughly chop the avocado, add to the chicken and pepper puree and combine, using a hand blender to make a slightly textured purée.

Tip Keep the pit in the unused avocado—this will reduce the discoloration.

Chicken, Leek, and Corn

Makes 1 serving

¼ **cup leek**
¼ **cup chicken breast, skinless**
2 **teaspoons olive oil**
⅓ **cup carrot**

¼ **cup potato**
  or sweet potato
2 **baby corn**
1 **tablespoon baby's usual**
  milk

Finely chop the leek, rinse the chicken and cut into small cubes. Heat the oil in a small saucepan and gently fry so the leek softens and the chicken cooks but does not brown. Check that the largest piece of chicken has cooked through.

Wash, peel, and dice or grate the carrot and sweet potato, dice the baby corn and stir into the pan. Add 1–2 tablespoons of water and the milk, cover, and simmer for 8 minutes.

Combine with a hand blender or push through a food mill to get the right consistency for your baby—as your baby becomes more confident, you will not need to blend.

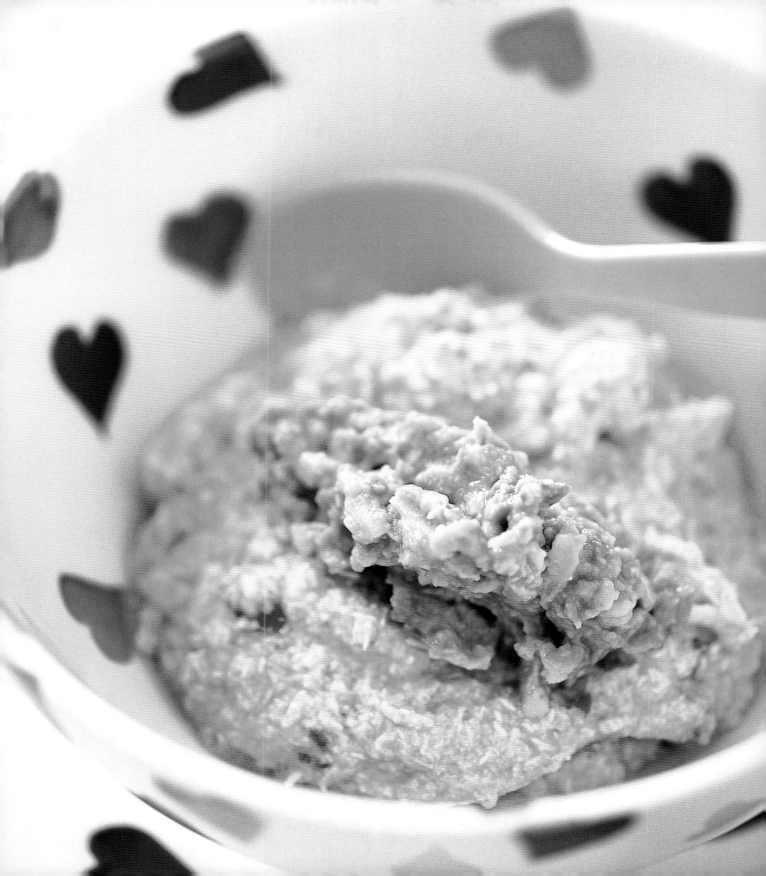

First Fish Stew

Makes 1 serving

2 tablespoons carrot
2 tablespoons potato
2 tablespoons rutabaga
2 tablespoons broccoli

1 sprig of fresh parsley
(optional)
2 tablespoons white fish
(skinless)

Wash and peel the carrot, potato, and rutabaga and grate or cut into $\frac{1}{8}$ inch dice. Wash and trim the broccoli and parsley (if using) and finely chop by hand or in the chopper attachment of a hand blender.

Wash the fish and cut into small cubes, removing any bits of bone. Put all the ingredients into a small saucepan and add just enough water to cover. Bring to a boil, then cover and reduce to a simmer for 12 minutes until the largest piece is soft and the fish flakes into the mixture. This can gently simmer for longer if you wish, bringing out the flavor as it reduces; just make sure to add enough water or a little of your baby's usual milk as needed.

Salmon, Broccoli, Cauliflower, and Potato Purée

A quick and easy way to introduce fish is to use a recipe you know your baby likes and mash in the steamed fish.
Makes 1 serving

½ cup broccoli
½ cup cauliflower
½ cup potato

1 ounce salmon, skinless

Follow the Broccoli, Cauliflower, and Potato Purée recipe on page 87 or defrost a pot of ready-made purée.

Rinse the salmon and dice into small cubes, checking as you cut for any small bits of bone. Steam for 8–10 minutes, making sure the largest piece is cooked right through.

Mash with a fork and stir into the purée, adding some of the steamer tray stock.

Tip The tail end of fish has less bone; explain when buying that it's for your baby and ask for some of the tail fillet.

Broccoli and Peas with Cheese

Your baby's first cheese experience—choose one that melts well such as cheddar or edam and don't forget mild, hard goat's cheese (chèvre).
Makes 1 serving

1/3 cup potato
1/2 cup broccoli

1/3 cup fresh or frozen peas
2 tablespoons mild hard cheese

Wash and peel the potato and trim and finely chop the broccoli. Bring 3 tablespoons of water to a boil and add the finely chopped broccoli, return to a boil, and reduce to a gentle simmer.

Dice the potato into 1/8 inch cubes or grate into the broccoli and add the peas. Cover and simmer for 10–12 minutes until all the pieces are soft.

Mash well or push through a food mill. While still hot, grate in the cheese and stir as it melts into the purée.

Eggy Mash

Most children love eggs, which is great because they are a nutritional marvel. Wait until 9 months—toward the end of stage 2—before you try this recipe. I've put Eggy Mash in this section because it's a very easy way to separate the white and yolk. Why? Some people are sensitive to the white and others to the yolk—so try Eggy Mash first with just the yolk as this is the least problematic, then the next time with just the white. If there is no reaction to either, you'll know that you're fine with the beaten-egg recipes in stage 3.

I would urge you to select organic free-range eggs, even if you are not convinced about organic the rest of the time.
Makes 1 serving

1/2 cup potato or sweet potato or 3–4 cubes of purée
1 egg—you will only need part of it

1 tablespoon of your baby's usual milk

Wash, peel, and chop the potato and steam or boil so that it is mashable.

Meanwhile hardboil an egg for 10 minutes, then remove and run under cold water until the egg is cool enough to peel. Peel and quarter the egg. Mash half the yolk or a quarter of the white in with the potato, adding the milk to make it creamy.

Serve at the right temperature for your baby in a morning or daytime feed, giving you the rest of the day to monitor any reactions.

Note Always make sure eggs are thoroughly cooked for a child under 12 months.

The first Christmas

Congratulations! This is your little darling's first Christmas, so make sure they're not feeling left out by giving them these festive treats.

Sweet Potato, Parsnip, Carrot, Onion, and Sage Mash

I prefer this steamed together as it seems to infuse the flavors—it can also be prepared by simmering together in a pan.

Makes 1 serving

¼ cup sweet potato
¼ cup parsnip
¼ cup carrot
1 tablespoon onion

2–3 sage leaves
A little of your baby's usual milk

Wash and peel the sweet potato, parsnip, carrot, and onion and grate or dice into ⅛ inch cubes. Rinse and chop the sage.

Mix together and steam for 10–12 minutes.

Mash with a little of your baby's usual milk and the stock from the steamer tray.

Plum and Prune Pudding

Not quite Christmas pudding but seasonal enough to feel that your baby is joining in their first Christmas celebration. Older kids not convinced by the delights of Christmas pudding may also like this as is or with yogurt or ice cream.

Makes 1 serving

3 ready-to-eat prunes, pitted
1 ripe plum or 2–3 cubes of plum purée

2 teaspoons millet flakes or fine oat flakes
Pinch of cinnamon (optional)

Chop the prunes into approximately ⅛ inch dice and simmer for 2 minutes in 2 tablespoons of water.

Peel the plum (see Peach, Plum, and Vanilla Purée on page 91) and remove the pit. Chop and add to the prunes and sprinkle in the millet or oat flakes and cinnamon, if using, stirring to avoid lumps.

Cook for 2–3 minutes, stirring frequently, until it thickens, then mix with a hand blender until it is the right consistency for your baby.

Week 6+: New Tastes and Nutritional Building Blocks

Some babies love variety, others prefer a more steady approach—it's fine to repeat one day's plan the following day, and you might find it easier to manage too. By the same token, remember to try out some new recipes now and then since it can be easy to get stuck in a favorite food rut. Remember to include a drink of water with mealtimes.

At this stage the principle is to introduce a protein-rich lunch. Particularly hungry babies may need a stop-gap between breakfast and lunch or as a dessert after dinner—a little yogurt and fruit purée is ideal.

The volume of breast or formula milk needed depends on age and weight, so vary accordingly.

	Wake-up	Breakfast	Lunch	Mid-afternoon	Dinner	Supper	Bedtime (optional)
Day 1	Breast milk or formula milk (1 cup)	No-gluten Muesli (see p.85)	Squash and Red Lentil Purée (see p.99) Kiwi, Prune, and Tofu Purée (see p.100)	Breast milk or formula milk (3/4 cup)	Potato, Parsnip, and Pear Purée (see p.87)	Breast milk or formula milk (3/4 cup)	Breast milk or formula milk (1/4 cup)*
Day 2	Breast milk or formula milk (1 cup)	Banana and Prune Purée (see p.84)	Chicken for Beginners (see p.104) Apple and Mango Purée (see p.96)	Breast milk or formula milk (3/4 cup)	Minty Pea and Potato Purée (see p.103)	Breast milk or formula milk (3/4 cup)	Breast milk or formula milk (1/4 cup)*
Day 3	Breast milk or formula milk (1 cup)	Millet and Fruits (see p.84)	Tofu, Fennel, and Spinach Purée (see p.100) Apple and Pear Purée (see p.96)	Breast milk or formula milk (3/4 cup)	Carrot and Sweet Potato Purée (see p.86)	Breast milk or formula milk (3/4 cup)	Breast milk or formula milk (1/4 cup)*
Day 4	Breast milk or formula milk (1 cup)	Beginner's Oatmeal (see p.84)	First Fish Stew (see p.106) Mango with Blackberry Ripple (see p.95)	Breast milk or formula milk (3/4 cup)	Broccoli, Cauliflower, and Potato Purée (see p.87)	Breast milk or formula milk (3/4 cup)	Breast milk or formula milk (1/4 cup)*
Day 5	Breast milk or formula milk (1 cup)	No-gluten Muesli (see p.85)	Chicken, Leek, and Corn (see p.104) Peach, Plum, and Vanilla Purée (see p.91)	Breast milk or formula milk (3/4 cup)	Pea and Bean Purée (see p.88)	Breast milk or formula milk (3/4 cup)	Breast milk or formula milk (1/4 cup)*
Day 6	Breast milk or formula milk (1 cup)	Banana and Prune Purée (see p.84)	Squash and Red Lentil Purée (see p.99) Quinoa, Rhubarb, and Vanilla Purée (see p.102)	Breast milk or formula milk (3/4 cup)	Spinach and Sweet Potato Purée (see p.88)	Breast milk or formula milk (3/4 cup)	Breast milk or formula milk (1/4 cup)*
Day 7	Breast milk or formula milk (1 cup)	Millet and Fruits (see p.84)	Salmon, Broccoli, Cauliflower, and Potato Purée (see p.106) Nectarine & Dried Apricot Purée (see p.92)	Breast milk or formula milk (3/4 cup)	Leek, Carrot, and Potato Purée (see p.88)	Breast milk or formula milk (3/4 cup)	Breast milk or formula milk (1/4 cup)*

* Optional, although many babies find it a comforting part of their bedtime routine

Stage three:
Independent weaning

They're beginning to become comfortable with feeding themselves.
This section is a pick 'n' mix selection of bite-size recipes they can get
their sticky paws into.

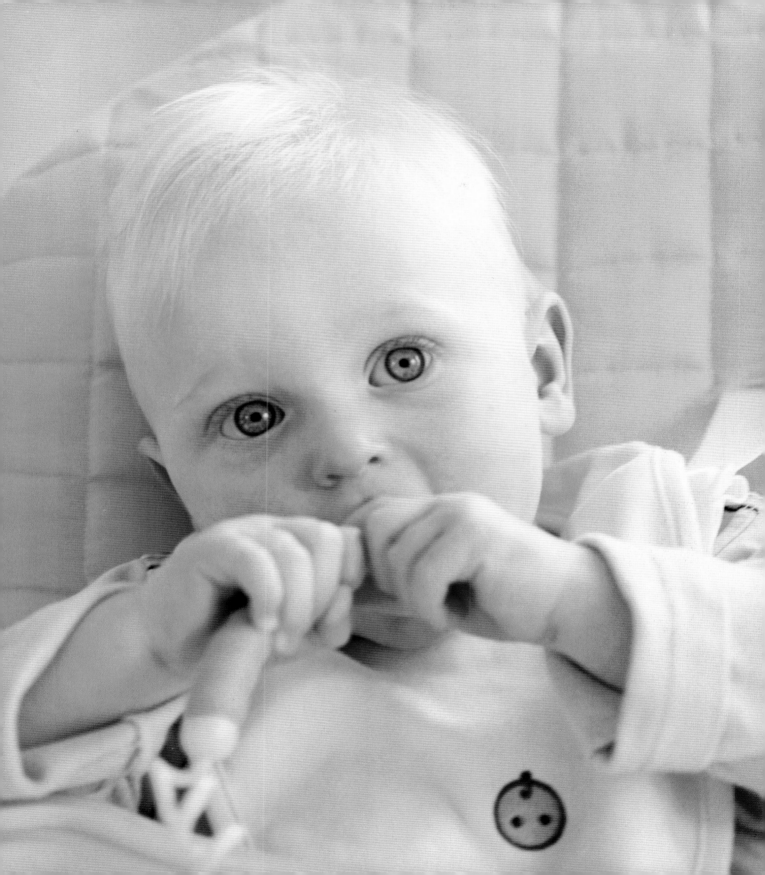

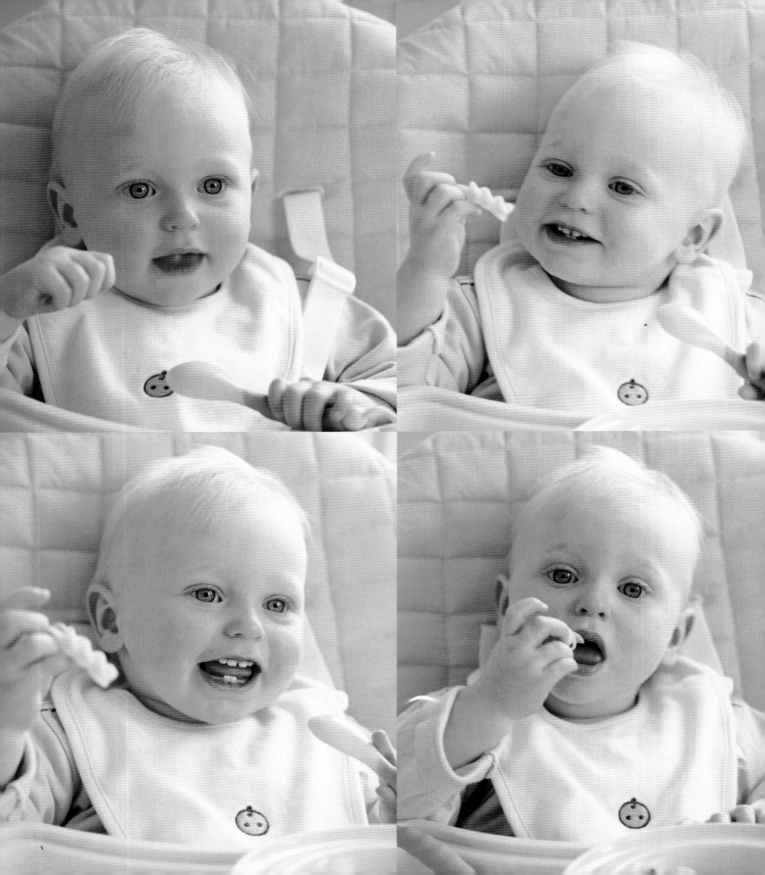

The third stage

Freedom, movement… and an opinion of their own. Your baby is changing daily and turning from a baby to a little person before your eyes. Their hand–eye coordination is developing at a rapid rate and so is their sense of cause and effect. Using cutlery is a huge step and you may find your little clever muffin will delight in trying to feed you (which is fair play, since you've been feeding them). It's time to swap those weaning spoons for child friendly cutlery, buying one set for your baby and one for you. Your baby should be 9–12 months old before you move onto this stage.

Letting your baby learn to feed themselves is a messy business. Cover the floor with a clean plastic mat that you can easily scrape food off (the mat needs to be cleaned and dried every time).

At this stage, their fingers seem to be picking up and feeling everything. It's no surprise that your baby will love finger food. After all, babies are sensual beings, and enjoying the sight, sound, and feel of food as much as the way it tastes is one of life's great pleasures. Finger foods help with the all-important skills of biting, chewing, and self-feeding. Remember to keep the food soft and an easy size to hold, making sure there are no seeds, pits, or bones. Relaxed finger food meals like sandwiches and pizza slices are easy for the evenings.

After a couple of months of eating more mashed food, your baby will be getting the hang of chewing, so it's time to introduce coarser bits. Even if your baby doesn't have many teeth, you'll be surprised how effective their gums are. The goal is slowly to introduce more solid, chewable foods until solid food is the main meal. Start with lightly cooked vegetables or bite-sized pieces of soft fruit. Next try raw, grated vegetables and finely chopped salads. Introduce new textures every two days and start to vary temperatures, serving some foods warm and others cold.

As your baby devours more solids, they'll drink less milk; if your baby isn't getting a taste for solids at this stage, it may be a good idea to reduce their milk intake slightly so that they're hungry for solids. Milk is still important, although much of their calcium can come from solid dairy products in foods like hard cheese, fromage frais, milk puddings, and yogurts. Remember, in order to digest calcium, your baby will need vitamin D, boron, magnesium, and manganese. While dairy is an important source of calcium, don't forget that nondairy sources, like broccoli, can have more. Other good sources of calcium include sardines, salmon, and egg yolks.

Your baby will now be enjoying three good meals a day and it's time to make them more adventurous. In a day, your baby should be eating around 3–4 servings of carbohydrates, at least 1 serving of a meat or fish protein or, if you're raising a vegetarian baby, 2 servings of a vegetable protein. A baby also needs 3–4 portions of fruit and vegetables, working up to the adult 5-a-day.

Start introducing foods with stronger flavors, like eggplant, mushrooms, pineapple, olives, and citrus fruits. Introduce them slowly and one at a time, so you can watch for any allergic reactions. You can also introduce wheat if you haven't already done so.

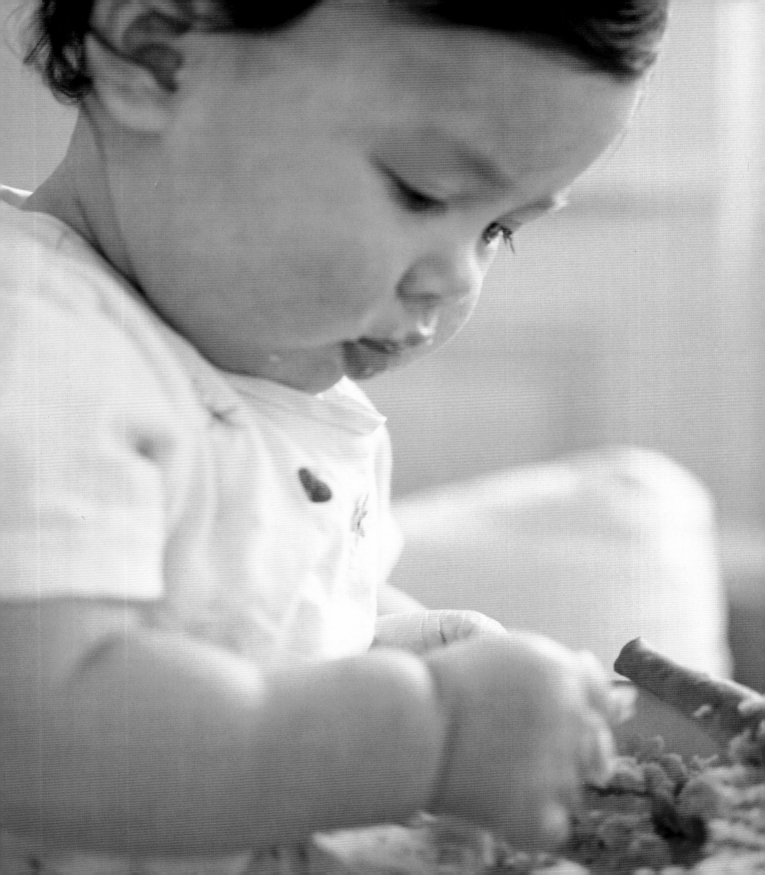

Mess and attitude

Your child is nearly walking or crawling and all of sudden they've got more attitude than Eminem. So what's the problem? Bottom line is that life's pretty frustrating at this age. Since they were born they've heard words, and slowly they should be starting to make sense of them. But as yet they can't quite get their message across. Their wah, nah, goo conversations will make perfect sense to them, but unfortunately not to you, so when you remove a toy or a doll, their verbal volley won't quite get the response they intend—so cue hysterical waterworks. They're probably used to having a small entourage, i.e. you, so don't be surprised if when you hand them over to Grandma, a friend, or a helper you get the serious diva treatment. They will also be prepared to put anything up their nose or down their throat, so make sure that small, round, or sharp objects—anything that could cause choking—are locked away in a secure cupboard or discarded.

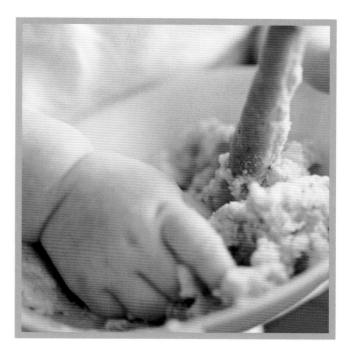

Be prepared

If you are the sort of person who likes everything neat, tidy, and in its correct place, take a deep breath now, because at this age everything goes out the window—quite often literally! Your child has an appetite for destruction and flinging a piece of food across the room and watching it slide down the fridge is damn good fun. If you're in the firing line don't take it personally. What was it Mom used to say?, "Patience is a virtue," so count to 3. It's not just food that will get the slam-dunk treatment—expect toys and cutlery to fly around, so don't give them the chance. If you're going to arm yourself with anything go for springy cutlery (see the photograph on page 111). This is a great invention because after attaching the suckers to their dining area, you can sit back and relax as they fling the cutlery away and it returns like a boomerang.

The most important thing to understand at this age is that your child is not trying to question your authority and doesn't have the cognitive ability to play mind games, so when they seemingly misbehave it's not a slight on you; it's just their way of expressing themselves. Try to enjoy this period because before you know it you'll have to deal with a real-life walking, talking living doll.

Choking

In cases of choking, follow the steps below:
- Do not attempt to retrieve the object with your fingers since this can push it further down the windpipe.
- Place your baby's head down along your forearm and give four sharp slaps across the top of the back between the shoulder blades. If this fails, turn the baby over and on to your lap. Give a few sharp thrusts on the lower breast bone using two fingers.
- If unsuccessful, repeat these measures and call emergency services.

Breakfast

Some independent babies become frustrated if they cannot feed themselves and you try to spoonfeed them. Try these recipes if your baby is insisting on finger foods or if you feel like adding some variety into their breakfast diet. Some of these recipes contain whole milk. Uncooked whole milk should not be given to babies under 12 months.

French Toast

Most French toast recipes add sugar and then smother with loads of honey or maple syrup. Honey is still a no-no until 12 months, so this recipe uses the natural sweetness of apple juice. Serve with bite-sized pieces of fresh fruit.

Makes approx. 20 cubes—enough for baby and 1 adult (not suitable for freezing)

1 medium egg
¼ cup apple juice
¼–½ teaspoon ground cinnamon
1 tablespoon butter

1 soft roll—preferably whole-wheat (to make your own, See No-salt Breadsticks dough recipe on page 126)
Selection of your child's favorite fresh fruit

Beat the egg until slightly fluffy. Add the apple juice and cinnamon and beat again.

Heat the butter in a nonstick skillet. Trim the bread roll of any hard or crispy crust and cut into bite-sized pieces (approx ¾ inch cubes).

Coat the bread cubes in the egg mixture (aim to coat rather than soak). Very fresh bread will take up the mixture quickly and go soggy, so try one cube first to test. Place the cubes in the skillet and cook until golden on each side.

Dust with a little extra cinnamon and serve with small size pieces of fresh fruit.

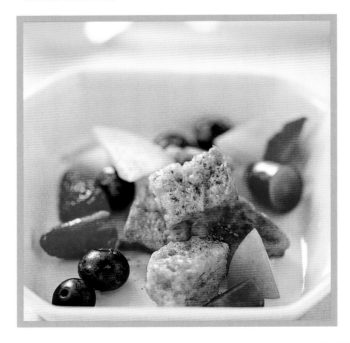

Plum and Oatmeal Pancakes

Finger food is easier than trying to manouver a spoon, but oatmeal as a finger food can start the day off in a sticky mess. This recipe is inspired by grown-up-style pancakes, but avoids using baking powder, which is too high in sodium for babies under 12 months (for older children a more traditional recipe can be found on page 145).

Makes 4 small pancakes /1–2 servings

(not suitable for freezing)

1 rounded tablespoon rolled oats

1 rounded tablespoon all-purpose flour

1 tablespoon whole milk

1 small plum, pitted (or other favorite fresh fruit)

1 tablespoon butter or margarine

1/2 medium egg*

Beat the rolled oats using the chopping attachment of a hand blender to form a coarse oat flour. Combine with the flour in a small mixing bowl and add the milk to form a thick batter. Wash and coarsely chop the plum (also works well with blueberries, banana, or apple).

Heat the butter in a large nonstick skillet.

Beat the egg until it has at least doubled in volume. When thick and stiff, fold into the oat batter, then finally stir through the fruit pieces.

Use a tablespoon to measure out the mixture for each pancake—they should spread to around 2 1/2 inches across. Cook on each side for 2 minutes until golden and cooked through.

Cut into small pieces as appropriate for your baby.

If you require a wheat-free version, replace the flour with an extra spoonful of oats (this will make a slightly heavier pancake).

*Rather than half an egg going to waste, double the quantities and make enough for the family. Although this recipe doesn't freeze, it will keep covered in the fridge for 24 hours—so simply toast or broil to reheat for the following day or as an after-school snack for older children or adults.

Cheese Dreams

Cheese Dreams was my grandma's grandiose name for eggy cheese sandwiches! They are similar to French toast—but savory.

Makes 1–2 servings (16 mini triangles)

(not suitable for freezing)

1 tablespoon butter

1 slice wholemeal bread

1/4 cup hard mild cheese

1 small egg

Freshly ground black pepper

Use a tiny amount of the butter to spread on the bread (it will help the sandwich stay together until the cheese melts). Slice the cheese and make a triangular sandwich with the bread and cut in half and half again until you have four mini triangles.

Beat the egg with the black pepper until slightly fluffy and heat the remaining butter in a non-stick frying pan. Dip the triangles in the egg to coat and slightly soak, then pan cook for 3 minutes on each side until golden, making sure the egg is thoroughly cooked and the cheese melted.

Stocks

Some recipes suggest using a stock, but commercial stock usually has added salt and can contain flavor enhancers. In particular, avoid stock cubes and powders that are both high in salt and contain monosodium glutamate (MSG). Stock is easy to make and can be made in batches and frozen in small pots or ice cube trays. It's handy as a base for soup, to gently flavor rice and to add depth of flavor to many recipes, but if time is not on your side all the recipes will work with water in place of the stock.

Basic Vegetable Stock

Makes about 2 pints

1 large carrot	**1 garlic clove (optional)**
$1/3$ cup leek	**1 bay leaf**
1 medium onion	**6 cups water**
$1/2$ cup celery	

Wash and roughly chop the vegetables and slice the garlic (this will give a milder taste than crushing).

Put all the ingredients in a large pan with the water and bring to a boil. Cover and simmer gently for about 1 hour. The volume of the stock will reduce by about a third, giving a greater intensity of flavor. Use a slotted spoon to remove the vegetable pieces, then push through a fine strainer. Cover and allow to cool, then freeze in small pots or ice cube trays.

Fish, Meat, or Poultry Stock

The leftovers from a roast are perfect for making stock—include any meat (but not fat) trimmings, but avoid skin that has been salted or seasoned.

Makes about 2 pints

1 large carrot	**6 cups water**
$1/3$ cup leek or 1 medium onion	**1–2 broiled trout carcass (bones and head) or cooked**
$1/2$ cup celery	**bones and meat trimmings**
1 bay leaf or sprig of fresh parsley	**(but not fat) from a roast**

Wash and chop the vegetables. Put all the ingredients in a large pan with the water and bring to a boil. Cover and simmer gently for about 1 hour until the volume of the stock reduces by about a third. If there is lot of fat on top of the stock, quickly drop in, then scoop out a couple of ice cubes (have a slotted spoon at the ready)—you will find that the fat clings to the cube and solidifies.

Remove the largest pieces with a slotted spoon then strain through a paper coffee filter or very fine strainer to make sure that no small bones end up in the finished stock. Cover and allow to cool, then freeze in small pots or ice cube trays.

Fish

Fish is a superb protein and contains calcium, magnesium, and selenium. Oily varieties, like mackerel, salmon, and tuna, are full of omega-3 and 6 fatty acids, crucial for brain development. Tuna scores high in the vitamin B^3, B^{12}, and D stakes, while salmon is full of potassium and magnesium. If buying fresh, choose fish that smells fresh not fishy; the eyes should look bright and clear and the flesh should be springy. Frozen fish is equally nutritious, and possibly fresher, if frozen at sea. If buying canned fish, choose fish packed in olive oil, sunflower oil, or water, not in brine.

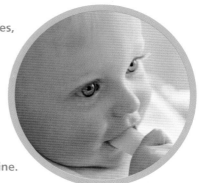

Eggy Herby Fish Bites

This recipe containing egg and salmon gives a double hit of brain-building omega–3.

Makes 1–2 servings (not suitable for freezing)

$^1/_4$–$^1/_2$ teaspoon mild fresh
   herbs (e.g. parsley, dill)
1 small egg
Small pinch of finely ground
   black pepper
1 teaspoon olive oil
$^1/_4$ cup skinless salmon or
   white fish

Wash and finely chop the herbs, then, in a small mixing bowl, beat into the egg and add the pepper.

Heat the oil in a nonstick skillet.

Wash and pat dry the fish with a kitchen towel, then cut into bite sized cubes, removing all bits of fish bone as you go. Put the fish in the egg mixture and coat thoroughly. Use a teaspoon to place the coated fish into the pan, making sure that there is a space between each piece to avoid clumping. Spoon any extra egg mixture over the fish pieces. Cook for 2–3 minutes on each side until browned and thoroughly cooked through.

For a simpler recipe, omit the herbs. Serve with rice or steamed potatoes.

Fisherman's Pie

Makes 1 serving

1 medium potato or sweet
   potato
2 teaspoons olive oil
$^1/_4$ cup onion or leek
$^1/_3$ cup skinned fish (white or
   salmon)
$^1/_4$ cup baby corn
$^1/_4$ cup carrots
$^1/_4$ cup peas
1 tablespoon water
1 tablespoon crème fraîche or
   $^1/_2$ tablespoon whole milk
2 teaspoons whole milk
1 tablespoon mild hard
   cheese, grated (optional)

Preheat the oven to 400°F. Wash, peel, and chop the potato and boil or steam until soft. Drain and set aside.

Heat the olive oil in a medium-sized saucepan. Finely chop the onion or leek and sauté.

Rinse the fish, check for bones, and chop into $^1/_2$ inch cubes. Chop the baby corn and carrot. Add the corn, carrot, peas, and fish to the onion and cook for 3 minutes. Stir in the water and crème fraîche.

Mash the potato with the milk.

Pour the fish mixture into a small ovenproof dish. Top with mashed potato and cheese. Bake for 20 minutes until the top is slightly browned. Serve.

Tuna Rice

Whether in sandwiches, pasta, or salad, tuna has become a staple of most adults' diets—oily fish is rich in vitamin B^{12}, D, omega-3, and, of course, protein. This recipe introduces tuna to your baby for the first time. It needs very little fish—so treat yourself to the rest in a salad or bake. Note, if using canned tuna, choose tuna packed in spring water or oil but not in brine because even when drained this will be too salty for your little one.

Makes 1 serving

(This recipe can be frozen, but cooked rice should not be stored at room temperature—use immediately once defrosted.)

2 tablespoons long-grain rice
1/4 cup fresh tuna (drained, if using canned; see note above)
1/4 cup zucchini
1/4 cup mushrooms
1/4 cup yellow or orange pepper
1/2 garlic clove, crushed (optional)
2–3 cherry tomatoes
1 teaspoon olive oil
1 teaspoon natural yogurt or whole milk (optional)

Steam or boil the rice until soft, drain and set aside.

If using fresh tuna, wash and chop the tuna. Then chop the zucchini, mushrooms, pepper, garlic, and tomatoes into 1/4 inch cubes. Steam the tuna and vegetables for 8 minutes. Alternatively, heat the oil in a small saucepan and gently cook the tuna with the garlic, if using. Add the vegetables and continue to cook for 3–4 minutes until the tuna is cooked through.

Stir in the rice, adding the milk or yogurt, if liked, to give a creamy finish.

Fish Creole

This mix of fruit, fish, and vegetables will become a firm favorite with children and grown-ups, especially for those who are not very enthusiastic about the flavor of fish on its own.

Makes 2–3 servings

1 tablespoon olive oil
1/2 medium onion (approx. 3 1/2 oz)
1 garlic clove
small piece fresh ginger (reduce to suit your child)
1 cup ripe tomatoes (or can of organic plum tomatoes)
1/2 cup fresh pineapple (or tinned in natural juice)
1/2 cup red pepper
1/3 cup green pepper
1/3 pound white fish, without skin or bones
Juice of 1 lime (optional)
Pinch of chili powder (optional)
Freshly ground black pepper

Warm the olive oil in a large skillet. Finely chop the onion, crush the garlic, and finely chop the ginger or crush (if you have a robust garlic press). Gently cook the onion, garlic, and ginger until the onion softens. Do not brown. Chop the tomatoes, pineapple, and peppers into bite-sized pieces and add to the onion, garlic, and ginger mix. Gently simmer for 5 minutes.

Wash and thoroughly check the fish for bones (you may find it useful to have a pair of kitchen tweezers to pull out the more stubborn bones).

Chop the fish into bite-sized chunks and add to the skillet. Either add 1 tablespoon of water or the lime juice, the chili powder, if using, and black pepper. Cover the pan and cook for 5–10 minutes until the fish is opaque and cooked through.

Serve with boiled rice or noodles.

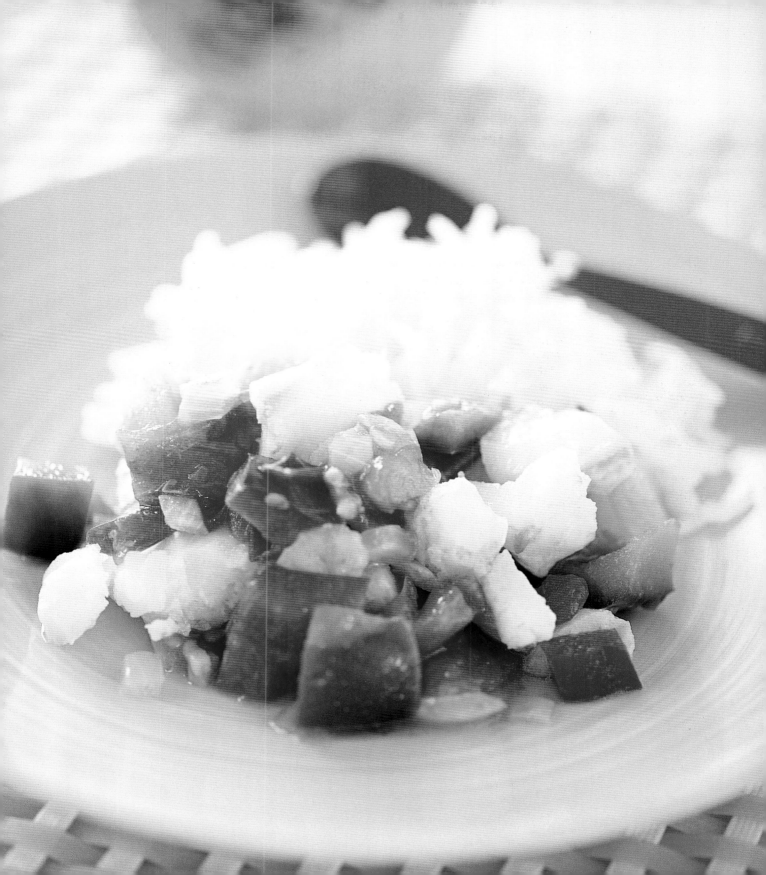

Chicken

A skinned, boned breast, which is the leanest part of the chicken, has less than half the fat of a steak. Chicken is a primary protein, packed with all eight essential amino acids as well as an abundance of vitamins A, B^3, B^6 and B^{12}. Choose organic chicken since free-range chickens may roam freely but can also be stuffed with hormones and antibiotics. Organic chickens are fed an organically grown diet and are able to wander about doing whatever chickens do.

Grandma Daisy's Casserole

It may be a bit extravagant to put the oven on for just one portion, so either prepare this when you have the oven on already, or multiply up and make a batch to freeze or feed the rest of the family.

Makes 1–2 servings

2 ounces skinless chicken breast or lean beef or lamb
1/4 cup leek
1 teaspoon olive oil or butter
1/2 cup carrot
1/2 cup potato
1/2 cup turnip or rutabaga
1/2 cup salt-free stock (see page 118) or water
1 small bay leaf (optional)
1 teaspoon parsley, chives, or thyme (optional)

Preheat the oven to 300°F.

Wash and dice the meat and cut into bite-sized cubes. Wash and slice the leek.

Heat the oil or butter in a small saucepan and cook the chicken and leek until they begin to brown. Place in a small ovenproof dish.

Wash, peel, and cube the carrot, potato and turnip or rutabaga and add to the chicken and leek mixture. Pour over the stock or water, sprinkle with the herbs and add the bay leaf, if using, and stir. Cover with foil and cook for 40 minutes to 1 hour. Stir halfway through, adding a little more water if needed. Remember to remove the bay leaf before serving.

Chicken Curry

Makes 1 serving

1 teaspoon olive oil
1/4 cup leek or onion
1 small garlic clove (optional)
2 ounces skinless chicken breast or ground chicken
1/4–1/2 teaspoon garam masala
1/4 cup carrot
1/3 cup potato
1/4 cup apple
4–5 golden raisins
1/4 cup salt-free stock (see page 118) or water

Heat the oil, finely chop the leek or onion, crush the garlic, if using, and add to the oil.

Rinse and cut the chicken into bite-sized cubes, sprinkle with the garam masala, and add to the pan. Stir until the chunks are cooked through.

Wash and peel the carrot, potato, and apple, and cut the raisins in half if necessary. Add to the pan, together with the stock and simmer for 10–15 minutes until the potatoes are cooked.

Sweet and Sour Chicken

Makes 1 serving

1 teaspoon olive oil
2–3 green onions
2 ounces skinless chicken
   breast
1/3 cup pak choi, green beans,
   or snow peas
1 small tomato

1/4 cup pineapple or mango
2–3 baby corn
1 tablespoon rice
1 tablespoon pineapple juice
2 tablespoons salt-free stock
   (see page 118) or water

Heat the oil in a nonstick skillet. Slice the green onions, cube the chicken, and add to the pan. Cook until slightly browned, then reduce to a low heat.

Wash and chop the vegetables and fruit and add to the pan. Increase the heat and bring back to a gentle simmer. Stir in the rice, juice, and stock and simmer until the rice is soft.

Tip For older children add a little tomato purée, Worcestershire sauce, or cider vinegar to bring out the sourness.

Chicken Bites

Makes 1–2 servings

2 teaspoons olive oil
1/2 egg, beaten
2 teaspoons cornstarch or
   whole-wheat flour

2 ou
breast

Heat the olive oil in a nonstick skillet. Beat the egg a gradually stir into the flour to form a simple batter.

Rinse and cut the chicken into bite-sized cubes. Dip the cubes in the batter and stir to coat.

Pan fry the chicken for about 2 minutes on each side until golden brown and both the egg and chicken are thoroughly cooked through.

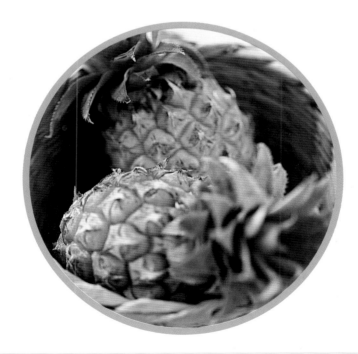

...ron and leads to tiredness, physical lethargy, and a lowered IQ. Since ...nd 6 months, this is something to be aware of. Enter iron-rich foods. ...d red by the myoglobin, an oxygen-storing pigment that houses ...nd therefore the more iron it will have. Red meat also has vast riches ...ample, contains more than the recommended daily allowance (RDA) ...nese, and selenium. When purchasing meat, look for lean, organic ...to nonorganic meats.

Makes 8 meatballs

2 ounces lean ground meat (beef, lamb, turkey or chicken)

1 tablespoon fresh whole-wheat breadcrumbs
2 tablespoons onion
1 teaspoon olive oil

Put the ground meat, breadcrumbs, and onion into the chopping bowl of a hand blender, and mix until smooth.

Measure out teaspoons of the mixture and roll into round, even, bite-sized balls.

Heat a teaspoon of olive oil in a nonstick skillet and gently fry the meatballs until brown. Serve with sauce (see page 125).

Tip If your child is not yet ready for whole meatballs, simply mash into the sauce with a fork

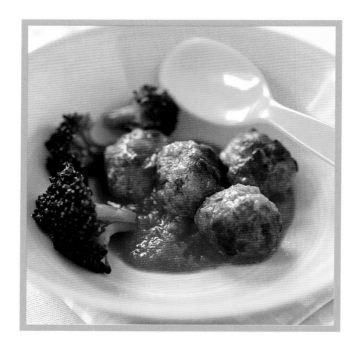

Meatball Sauce

Makes 2–3 servings

1 teaspoon olive oil
2 tablespoons red onion
1/4 cup carrot
1/4 cup sweet potato
1/4 medium fresh beet or 1
   tablespoon beet purée
   (page 66)

1–2 tablespoons water
1/4 cup red pepper
1 small ripe tomato 2
   teaspoons whole milk

Heat the olive oil in a small saucepan. Finely chop the onion and gently cook.

Wash, peel, and finely chop the carrot and sweet potato (if using fresh beet, peel and finely chop and add here) and add to the onion. Cook for a further 3 minutes, then add the water and gently simmer.

Wash and chop the red pepper and tomato and add to the pan together with the milk. Bring to a boil and simmer for a further 4 minutes. If using beet purée, stir through a little at a time to color the sauce to the desired red. Purée with a hand blender until it is the appropriate texture for your child.

Quick meatball sauce method: if you have frozen cubes of purées, simply sweat the onion with the olive oil and add a frozen cube each of carrot and sweet potato purée, and 1 cube of beet purée. Heat until defrosted. Wash and finely chop the tomato and red pepper and stir in with the milk (and, if needed, additional water). Blend as before.

Goulash

The traditional Hungarian recipe typically has lashings of paprika and cayenne pepper. This is somewhat milder although quite a lot of young children enjoy a bit of spice—especially if breastfed by a mom who loves spicy foods. Vary the quantities to suit the preference of your child.

This recipe introduces eggplant—as with all new foods, try a little first to check for any allergic reaction before making up large batches.

Makes 1 serving

2 ounces lean beef, lamb, or
   chicken
1/2 small onion
1 teaspoon olive oil
1/4 cup green pepper
1/4 cup eggplant
1 small ripe tomato
1 garlic clove

Large pinch of paprika
A little freshly ground black
   pepper
1/2 cup salt-free stock (see
   page 118)
1 tablespoon rice
Pinch of cayenne pepper
   (optional for an older child)

Chop the meat into bite-sized cubes and finely chop the onion.

Heat the olive oil in a saucepan and slightly brown the meat with the onion. Wash, chop, and add all the other ingredients except the stock and rice and stir continuously until they start to sizzle. Pour in the stock and rice, bring to a boil, and simmer, stirring occasionally, until the rice is soft, adding a little more stock or water if needed.

For an older child, add a little pinch of cayenne pepper and more paprika before adding the rice.

Taking a dip

Using raw vegetables or a breadstick may not seem such a major step, but for a baby this is one giant leap into the world of cutlery and eating like an adult. Also these recipes save on cooking time if you have friends coming around.

No-salt Breadsticks

Breadsticks are handy for dipping into sweet and savory purées and are a good way to introduce a child to the idea of cutlery. They also make great teething sticks for your baby.

The same dough recipe can be used as a pizza base as well as rolls for burgers and buns.

Makes approx. 40 breadsticks

¾ **cup strong whole-wheat flour**
1 **teaspoon dried yeast (most fast-acting yeasts do not require sugar to be added—read the instructions on the** envelope to check and add accordingly)
½ **cup hand-hot water**
2 **teaspoons olive oil**

Preheat the oven to 425°F.

Combine the flour and yeast in a mixing bowl. Pour in the water and oil and use your fingers to make a dough.

Lightly flour a clean work surface and knead for 5 minutes. Divide the mix into two, cover half with a lightly oiled piece of plastic wrap to prevent it drying out and set aside. Roll the remaining dough into a long sausage approximately ¼ inch in diameter and cut into short breadstick lengths (approx. 2¾ inches).

Lay on a lightly oiled baking sheet and bake for 20–25 minutes until golden and crisp (they should not be soft since they will not keep). Repeat for the remaining dough.

Allow to cool and store in an airtight container for up to 1 week.

Baby-friendly Hummus (Chickpea Purée)

Chickpeas may be small, but they're a rich source of protein, carbohydrate, B-group vitamins, and monounsaturated fats. They are digested slowly so help to stabilize blood sugar levels and aid the slow release of sugar into the bloodstream. They are also perfect for parents bringing up their babies on a vegan or vegetarian diet.

Hummus is traditionally made with tahini—a sesame-seed-based paste, but it is best to wait until your child is older before giving them seeds. Store-bought hummus can also be high in salt and other additives. This simplified hummus is a great dipping purée since it's sticky enough to stay put on the breadsticks or crudités.

½ **medium onion**
1–2 **garlic cloves (depending on the taste of your child)**
1–2 **tablespoons olive oil**
¾ **cup chickpeas (canned in water, not brine)**
Juice of ¼ **lemon or lime**
(optional)
¼ **teaspoon paprika** (optional)

Finely chop the onion and crush the garlic. Heat 1 tablespoon of olive oil in a nonstick skillet and gently cook the onion and garlic until soft but not brown. Drain and rinse the chickpeas and combine with the onion, garlic, and optional extras in the chopping attachment of a hand blender. Blend until smooth. Add a little additional olive oil and a tablespoon of water to create a smooth glossy paste.

Serve with breadsticks and baby-sized crudités.

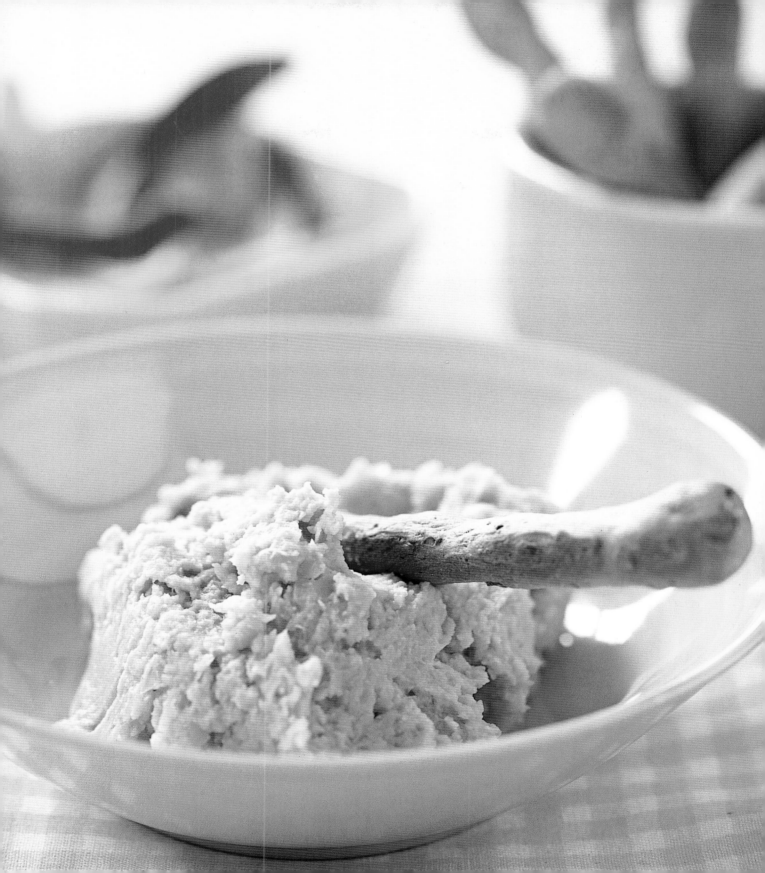

Cheesy Broccoli, Cauliflower, and Potato Dip

Makes 1 serving

1 portion of Broccoli, Cauliflower, and Potato Purée (see page 87)

2–3 tablespoons mild hard cheese

If using frozen purée, defrost and heat in a saucepan or microwave. Grate the cheese and stir in until melted. Serve with No-salt Breadsticks (see page 126).

Most of the stage 2 purées can also be used as dips just as they are or add herbs, grated cheese, or a little natural yogurt for variety.

Avocado Dip

Makes 1 serving

¼–½ ripe avocado

1 tablespoon natural yogurt

Simply mash the avocado into the yogurt and serve with No-salt Breadsticks (see page 126) and steamed crudités (see right).

Herby Crème Fraîche with Steamed Crudités

Makes 1 serving

1–2 teaspoons fresh herbs, e.g. mint, chives, basil, dill
1 tablespoon crème fraîche (or natural yogurt)
For the crudités choose a colorful selection from:
½ small carrot
Small stalk of celery

1–2 small broccoli or cauliflower florets
2–3 snow peas
2–3 baby corn
¼ cup cucumber
½ small parsnip
2–3 string beans

Wash then very finely chop the herbs and stir through the crème fraîche. When your child is more confident with finger food, most of the crudités can be eaten raw, but in the meantime wash and cut into small sticks or batons and steam for 2–3 minutes to soften. They can be eaten warm or chilled, covered, and stored in the refrigerator for up to 12 hours.

Fruit Dips

You can dip fruit in breakfast purées, fruit purées, yogurts, and fromage frais.
Makes 1 serving

Think rainbow colors when you select from:
½ small banana
¼ cup mango
¼ cup papaya (paw paw)
½ peach
½ nectarine

½ apple
½ pear
3–4 grapes (seedless and halved)
½ kiwi fruit
1–2 dried apricots or prunes (gently boiled until soft)

If the fruit is very ripe, simply cut into baby-sized batons, otherwise lightly steam until tender.

To sweeten natural yogurt , stir through a little apple juice, pineapple juice, or cook and strain a few raspberries (removing the seeds). See also Frozen Fruit Sticks on page 134.

Vegetable treats

The following recipes are simple, easy introductions to proper meals. I've given you a range of tastes and textures to choose from and a couple of quick options (Bean Bites and My First Pizza) that will feed the baying masses in a moment.

Moroccan Couscous

Traditionally this is a combination of spicy fruit and vegetables with couscous (made from durum wheat). The recipe will also work well with quinoa instead of couscous. Make sure that you cook it until the grain is soft.
Makes 1–2 servings

1/2 **cup vegetable stock (see page 118) or water**
2 **tablespoons couscous**
2 **dried apricots**
1 **teaspoon olive oil**
2 **green onions**
1/4 **cup red pepper**
1 **tablespoon peas (fresh or frozen)**
1 **garlic clove**

1/4 **cup butternut squash purée (see page 64)**
1/4 **teaspoon finely chopped fresh cilantro or small pinch of dried cilantro**
1/4 **teaspoon cumin**

Heat the stock in a medium saucepan. Rinse the couscous and chop the dried apricots and stir into the stock. Reduce the heat and gently simmer for 5–10 minutes to soak and soften.

Heat the oil in a nonstick skillet. Finely chop all the other ingredients and sauté, adding the butternut squash purée toward the end to heat through as well as the herbs and cumin.

Mix in the couscous and apricots and serve as is or purée slightly with a hand blender to suit your child.

If your child is over 12 months old and not allergic to nuts, try adding a few finely chopped cashews.

Cheesy Risotto

Traditionally risotto is made by gradually adding liquid to the rice, allowing the liquid to be soaked up by the rice before adding more. This is a simplified method—not traditional but practical.
Makes 1–2 servings

1 **teaspoon olive oil**
1/4 **cup leek**
1/4 **cup zucchini (also works well with broccoli, peas, string beans, or fennel)**
1/4 **cup red or yellow pepper**
1/4 **cup butternut squash or red kuri**
Large pinch of dried oregano

2 **tablespoons wild, brown, or risotto rice**
1/2 **cup vegetable stock (see page 118) or water**
3 **tablespoons hard cheese**

Heat the oil in a medium saucepan. Wash and finely chop the leek, zucchini, pepper, and squash and add to the pan with the oregano. Stir well and gently cook for 2 minutes.

Rinse the rice and stir into the mixture, coating the grains, then stir in the stock. Bring to a boil, then reduce to a gentle simmer. Cover the pan and cook for 20 minutes until the rice is soft, stirring occasionally. Grate the cheese into the mixture, then melt in. Allow to cool to the right temperature for your baby and serve.

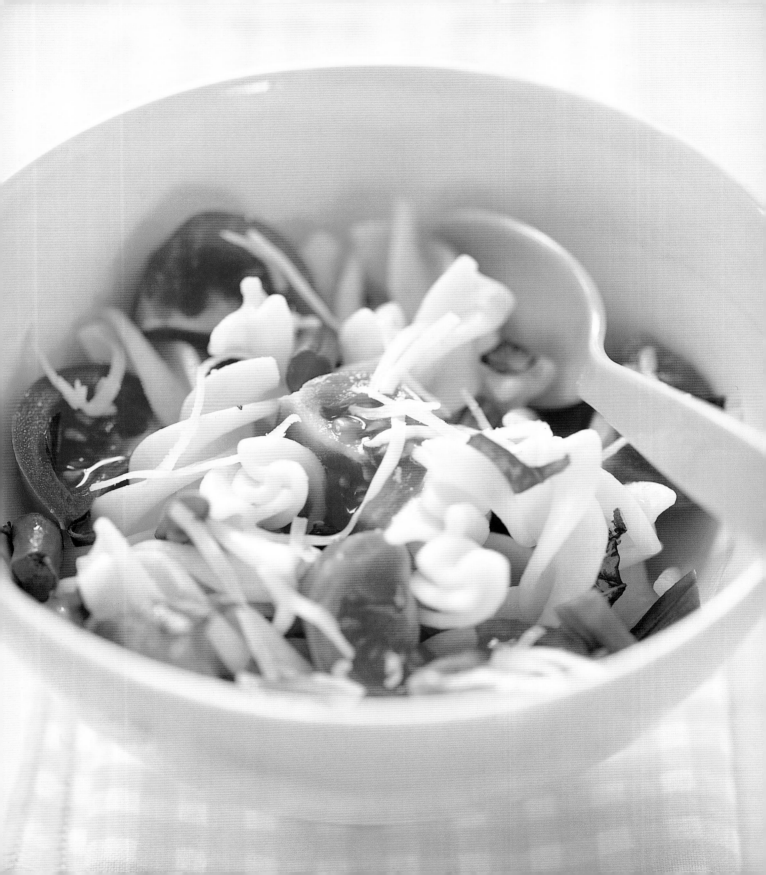

Tricolore Cold Pasta Salad

This cold salad is ideal for the child who wants to feed themselves and is able to chew. They will enjoy the mix of textures in finger-food-size pieces. For a less confident weaner use tiny soup pasta and cook, then blend in the other ingredients with a hand blender to make a fresh-tasting sauce.
Makes 1–2 servings

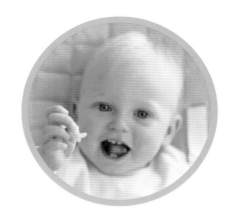

2 tablespoons pasta shapes
3 cherry tomatoes
3 tablespooons snow peas

3 tablespoons hard mild cheese, grated
Few fresh basil leaves (optional)

Cook the pasta following the instructions on the package. Cut the cherry tomatoes in quarters and slice the snow peas into bite-size pieces. If your child is not yet able to chew confidently, steam the tomato and snow peas for 5 minutes until tender, otherwise leave raw.

Drain the pasta and rinse with cold water.

Combine all the ingredients and serve.

My First Pizza

Makes 4 baby pizzas

No-salt Dough (see page 126)
16 cherry tomatoes (4 per pizza)

1/2 cup mild hard cheese per pizza
Fresh basil leaves (optional)

Preheat the oven to 425°F.

Shape the dough 3 1/4 inch diameter disks and place on a lightly oiled baking sheet.

Slice the cherry tomatoes into three and arrange on the dough disks. Grate the cheese and sprinkle on each. Bake for 15–20 minutes until the cheese begins to brown and the base is cooked but not hard.

Allow to cool and serve one with a sprinkle of chopped basil, if using. Freeze the others in individual bags.

Lentil, Fennel, and Tofu

Makes 1–2 servings

1/2 cup vegetable stock (see page 118) or water
3 tablespoons dried red lentils
1/4 cup potato
1/4 cup fennel bulb
1/4 cup firm tofu

1/4 cup red pepper
1/4 cup broccoli or green beans
1/4 teaspoon fresh parsley or chives

Bring the stock or water to a boil, reduce to a simmer, and cover. Check the lentils for any grit or chaff and rinse thoroughly. Stir into the stock and continue to simmer for 15 minutes, adding more water if needed.

Wash, peel, and chop the potato and add to the simmering lentils. Wash and shred the fennel, drain then cube the tofu, rinse and slice the pepper and broccoli, and finely chop the herbs. Add to the stock, bring to a boil, and return to a gentle simmer for 5–10 minutes until the potato and lentils are soft. Allow to cool and serve.

Fruity Bean Pilaf

Use canned beans rather than cooking from dried, but choose beans that are canned in water rather than sugared water or brine. Kidney beans, in particular, require very careful cooking from dried—if you do decide to go this route, follow the package instructions very carefully.

Makes 1 serving

1/4 cup mixed beans
1 medium tomato
1 dried apricot
1 teaspoon golden raisins
2 tablespoons brown rice
1 garlic clove

2 tablespoons corn
1/2 cup vegetable stock (see page 118) or water
1/4 teaspoon garam masala

Rinse and chop the beans, tomato, apricot, and golden raisins (if necessary).

Rinse and drain the rice and crush the garlic. Combine all the ingredients in a saucepan and bring to a boil, cover, and reduce to a simmer. Cook for 20 minutes, stirring occasionally, until the rice is soft.

Allow to cool and serve.

Green Thai Tofu

This deliciously fragrant recipe includes creamed coconut. Coconut is not a high allergy risk, even though it is technically a nut, and it is extremely rare for anyone, even with a nut allergy, to react to coconut. Even so, as when introducing all new foods to your baby, start by making a small quantity early in the day to give you a chance to monitor any adverse reactions.

Makes 1 serving

1–2 teaspoons olive oil
1 green onion
1/2 inch cube fresh ginger
1 inch lemongrass (optional)
1/3 cup potato
1/4 cup carrot
1/4 cup spinach or broccoli
2–3 button mushrooms

3–4 string beans
1/2 cup vegetable stock (see page 118) or water
1/2 teaspoon fresh cilantro
1/4 cup firm tofu
1 tablespoons creamed coconut or 1 tablespoon milk

Heat the oil in a nonstick skillet. Slice the green onion diagonally into strips, peel and grate the ginger, and sauté with the lemongrass, if using.

Wash the other vegetables, peel and chop the potato and carrot into small cubes, tear the spinach and slice the mushrooms and beans. Add to the pan. Cook for 2 minutes to release the flavors but do not brown. Stir in the stock, bring to a boil and simmer. Finely chop the cilantro and add to the pan. Cook for 5 minutes.

Drain the tofu and cut into small cubes and grate the creamed coconut, stir into the pan, and simmer for another 8 minutes until the potato and carrot are soft.

Remember to remove the piece of lemongrass before serving. Allow to cool before serving.

Bean Bites

Many vegetarian dishes for this age tend to be wet stews and casseroles—not so great if your child loves finger food. Small bean burgers can be eaten warm or cold.

Makes 8–12 bean bites

½ cup tinned mixed beans
¼ cup sweet potato
3 tablespoons leek
2 teaspoons cornstarch

¼ teaspoon fresh herbs
   (optional)
¼–½ egg, beaten
2–3 teaspoons olive oil

Rinse the beans and wash, peel and coarsely chop the sweet potato and leek. Put all the ingredients except the egg and olive oil into the chopping attachment of a hand blender and purée until smooth (the mixture may be quite dry, so you may not manage a completely smooth result).

Beat the egg and gradually add to the mixture, using at least a quarter of the egg until the consistency resembles that of hummus.

Heat half the oil in a nonstick skillet, then, using a teaspoon, drop blobs of the mixture into the pan, making sure that there's a little space between each one to prevent them sticking together. Cook for 4–5 minutes, drizzling in a little more oil as needed. Flip with a spatula, check the underside is golden, and cook for a further 4–5 minutes. Serve with steamed or raw crudités and dips.

Lentil Casserole

Makes 1–2 servings

1 cup vegetable stock (see
   page 118) or water
3 tablespoons dried red lent
½ cup butternut squash or
   rutabaga
¼ cup potato

herbs

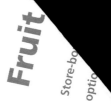

Heat the stock in a medium saucepan. Rinse the lentils, checking over for any small grit, and stir into the stock. Wash, peel, and coarsely chop all the vegetables and stir into the stock, adding the herbs. Bring to a boil, then either reduce to a gentle simmer, cover and cook for 30 minutes, stirring occasionally, or, if you have the oven on, pour into a small casserole dish, cover, and bake at 300°F for 20–25 minutes.

and desserts

Store-bought desserts can be a bit of a minefield of sugar and preservatives, so I've included these healthy, natural options that are reasonably worthy but shouldn't send your child running to the hills in disgust.

Frozen Fruit (and Vegetable) Sticks

Gums can be very painful during these months with teething in full swing. Once your child is able to hold and chew a piece of fruit or a breadstick, this simple method will enable you to freeze hand-sized fruit sticks that will not only soothe sore gums, but also encourage your baby to eat more fruit and vegetables.

Choose from:	Plum
Apple	Carrot
Peach	Butternut squash
Nectarine	Sweet potato

Wash, peel, and cut your chosen fruit and vegetables into baby-sized sticks.

Steam the vegetables for 6–8 minutes to soften. Leave to cool.

To prevent the sticks ending up as a large clump, lay the sticks on a baking sheet (checking first that it will fit in your freezer), making sure there is space between each one. Freeze for 1 hour, then transfer into small freezer bags. When required allow the sticks to warm up a little—if you give them to your child straight from the freezer, they can be too cold and freeze burn (if in doubt check one yourself first).

Hint Older children will love these too, especially in summer when you can include berries. Serve on their own or with yogurt.

Apple Cinnamon Crumble Pot

Little ovenproof ramekin dishes are perfect for making these individual crumble pots. See the Oaty Crumble recipe on page 50 for ideas on how to spice it up and add ingredients for an adult version.
Makes 1 serving

½ apple or 3–4 cubes apple purée (see page 70)	Pinch of cinnamon
1 teaspoon golden raisins (chopped if large)	1 dessertspoon oats
	1 tablespoon butter (very cold)

Preheat the oven to 400°F.

Wash, peel, and chop the apple and cook with a little water in a small saucepan (or melt the frozen purée). Stir in the raisins and cinnamon and simmer for 3–4 minutes. Pour into the ramekin.

Put the oats in the chopping bowl of a hand blender and grate in the butter. Blend until they resemble breadcrumbs and sprinkle onto the apple mixture. Bake for 15 minutes until slightly golden. Leave to cool a little before serving.

This recipe works well with most other fruit, although if made with banana it will not freeze well.

Real Fruit Gelatin

Most store-bought Jello is high in artificial colors and flavors, but it is surprisingly easy to make your own fruit desserts with either gelatin or the vegetarian alternative, agar agar. Some fruits are too acidic and won't set however hard you try, for example kiwi fruit, and some require cooking first (see below) because they contain an enzyme that will prevent them from setting. Choose powdered gelatin or agar agar in preference to leaves.

Makes 2 servings

2 heaped teaspoons
   powdered gelatin or agar
   agar
2¼ cups juice made up of one
   or more of the following:
Apple
Pear
Grape
Red- or blackcurrant
Blackberry
Raspberry

**The following are brought to
   a boil for 5 minutes before
   adding the gelatin or agar
   agar:**
Pineapple
Mango
Papaya
Peach
Nectarine

If making the juices yourself, wash the fruit and bring to a boil in a little water until soft, then strain to remove skins and seeds etc. Make up to 2¼ cups by adding extra apple juice for sweetness.

Put the juice in a clean saucepan, bring to a boil, and simmer, then sprinkle in the gelatin or agar agar, stirring continuously until fully dissolved.

Put some cold water on to a saucer and drip a couple of drops of the mixture on to the water to check it is strong enough to set—it should form a jelly blob. If not, sprinkle in a little more gelatin or agar agar and repeat. If it goes very thick, add a little more apple juice.

Pour into molds, or small glass dishes, cool and refrigerate until set (takes about 3 hours).

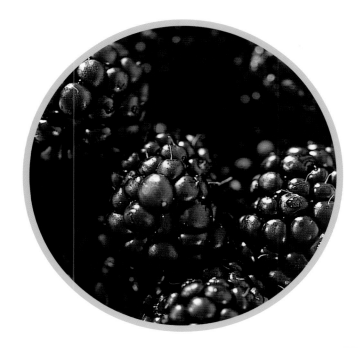

Christmas dinner treats

Christmas is the time of a few extra drinks, a few extra sweet treats, and a few sneaky kisses under the mistletoe, and your child will want to be part of festive activities as they feed on your anticipation of the upcoming event. While overindulging them isn't wise and buying presents is a bit pointless since the wrapping paper will be far more enticing than the gift itself, there is a way to treat your child. Grab the high chair, make them the center of attention at the table, and serve these treats at the same time as the main meal. They'll just love being part of the big dinner extravaganza!

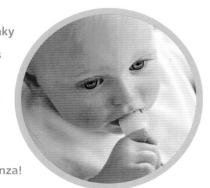

Turkey Christmas Dinner

Makes 1 serving

2 ounces turkey breast
¹/₄ cup carrot
¹/₄ cup parsnip
¹/₄ cup potato or sweet potato
3 tablespoons leek
¹/₄ cup broccoli or 1 Brussels sprout
2–3 fresh sage leaves or pinch of dried sage

Rinse the turkey breast and chop into ¹/₄–¹/₂ inch cubes. Steam the turkey and meanwhile wash and peel the vegetables and chop into ¹/₄–¹/₂ inch cubes. Add the vegetables with the sage to the turkey and steam for a further 5 minutes until the turkey is thoroughly cooked and the vegetables are soft (the turkey should be steamed for 10–12 minutes in total).

Serve as is to a confident independent weaner with the collected steamer stock, or mix with a hand blender to a chunky purée.

My First Christmas Pudding

Traditional Christmas pudding is too rich (and alcoholic!) to give to a young child—here's a simplified version. It is delicious as it is or serve with a swirl of natural yogurt.

Makes 1 serving

2 prunes (pits removed)
2–3 dried apricots (sulfur-free, pits removed)
1 teaspoon golden raisins or raisins
¹/₄ cup apple
¹/₄ cup carrot
1 tablespoon oats
Large pinch of mixed spice, e.g. cinnamon, ginger
1 tablespoon whole milk

Roughly chop the prunes and apricots, removing any bits of pit. Put in a saucepan with the raisins and enough water to cover them and bring to the boil.

Wash, peel, and grate the apple and the carrot and add to the dried fruit. Simmer for 1 minute. Stir in the oats and spices with the milk and a little extra water if needed. Cover, bring back to a boil and simmer for 8–10 minutes, stirring occasionally.

From 9 months: Independent Weaning

Milk is still important; however, by this stage guidelines recommend no more than 18fl oz–1 pint per day, although the planner does not specify how this should be spread across the day—vary to suit your child.

Fruit and vegetables are important. Keep a lidded plastic container in the fridge with a selection of fruit and vegetable sticks and dried fruit as handy snacks between meals—the coolness will also soothe sore gums.

Your baby will enjoy learning to feed himself, but never leave a baby alone with cutlery or finger foods.

Remember to include a drink of water with mealtimes.

	Wake-up	Breakfast	Lunch	Mid-afternoon	Dinner	Supper	Bedtime (optional)
Day 1	Breast milk or formula milk	No-gluten Muesli (see p.85) with Fruit Dips (see p.128)	Chicken Curry (see p.122) with broccoli florets or green beans Peach, Plum, and Vanilla (see p.91)	Breast milk or formula milk	Broccoli and Peas with Cheese (see p.107) Banana and Prune Purée (see p.84)	Breast milk or formula milk	Breast milk or formula milk *
Day 2	Breast milk or formula milk	Plum and Oatmeal Pancakes (see p.117)	Fish Creole (see p.120) with rice or noodles Pear, Raisin, and Sultana Purée (see p93)	Breast milk or formula milk	No-salt Breadsticks (see p.126) with Dips (see p.128) Yogurt or fromage frais	Breast milk or formula milk	Breast milk or formula milk *
Day 3	Breast milk or formula milk	Beginner's Oatmeal (see p84) with Fruit Dips (see p.128)	Mini Meatballs in Meatball Sauce (see pp.124–5) with broccoli florets Fresh fruit pieces	Breast milk or formula milk	Cheesy Risotto (see p.129) Apple and Mango Purée (see p.96)	Breast milk or formula milk	Breast milk or formula milk *
Day 4	Breast milk or formula milk	French Toast (see p.116)	Green Thai Tofu (see p.132) Strawberry and Banana Mash (see p.93)	Breast milk or formula milk	My First Pizza (see p.131) Real Fruit Jelly (see p.135)	Breast milk or formula milk	Breast milk or formula milk *
Day 5	Breast milk or formula milk	No-gluten Muesli (see p.85) with Fruit Dips (see p.128)	Bean Bites (p.133 or p.119, p.123) with Eggy Mash (see p.107) Fruit Dips (see p.128)	Breast milk or formula milk	Tricolore Cold Pasta Salad (see p.131) Mango with Blackberry Ripple (see p.95)	Breast milk or formula milk	Breast milk or formula milk *
Day 6	Breast milk or formula milk	Cheese Dreams (see p.117)	Grandma Daisy's Casserole (see p.122) Fresh fruit pieces	Breast milk or formula milk	Herby Crème Fraîche with Crudités (see p.128) Apple Cinnamon Crumble Pot (see p.134)	Breast milk or formula milk	Breast milk or formula milk *
Day 7	Breast milk or formula milk	Beginner's Oatmeal (see p84) with Fruit Dips (see p.128)	Fisherman's Pie (see p.119) Yogurt or fromage frais	Breast milk or formula milk	Lentil, Fennel and Tofu (see p.131) Nectarine and Dried Apricot Purée (see p.92)	Breast milk or formula milk	Breast milk or formula milk *

* Optional, although many babies find it a comforting part of their bedtime routine.

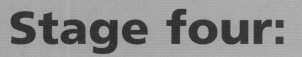

Stage four:
Toward adult food

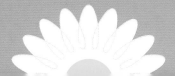

This section provides healthy, easy-to-prepare, toddler meals as well as tips on introducing difficult vegetables (including a recipe on how to make Cabbage Ice Cream!).

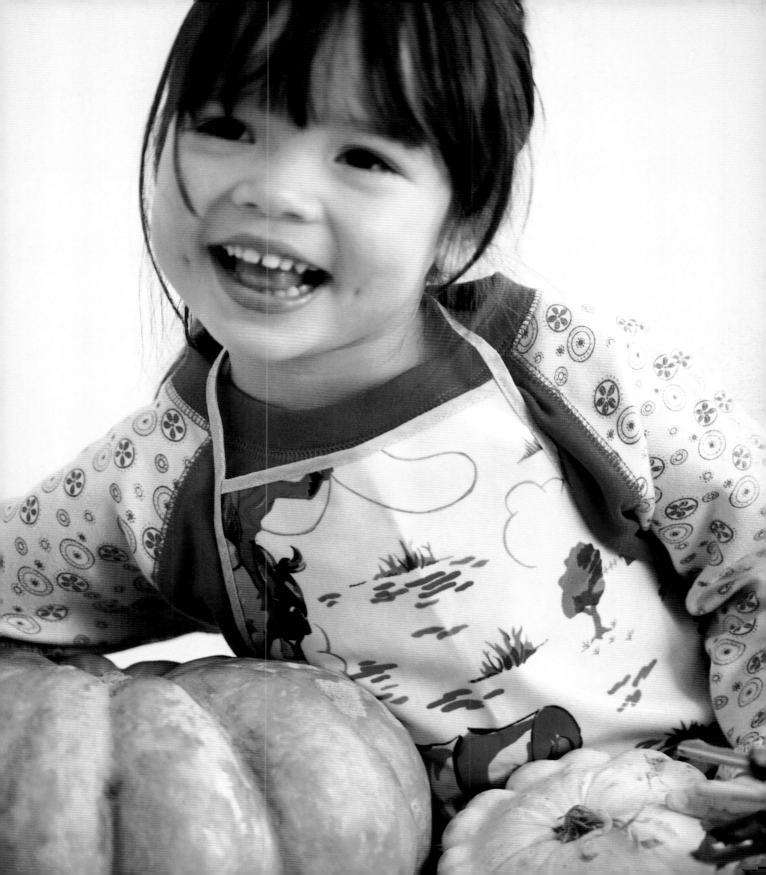

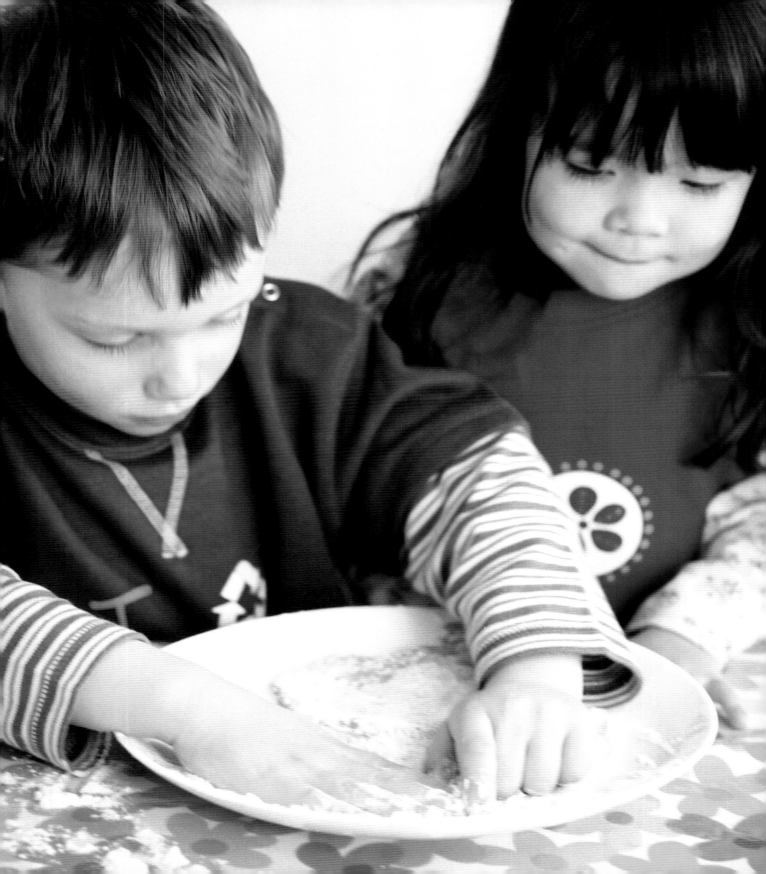

The fourth stage

This section includes more meal ideas but also deals with areas where you may be struggling to get your child to eat. Stage 4 meals are for 12 months and on, but remember to include stage 3 meals and increase the portions.

Toddler meals

As a toddler's tastebuds go on the magical mystery tour of discovery, you'll find their choices will be as wide and varied as Elton John's back catalogue. Some children don't like to see what they're eating, while others need to have every food displayed on their plate. Some children will like fantasy foods (just rename a dish "Bob the Builder's oatmeal"), while others simply want to get stuck in. Some children will like three big sit-down meals with a few snacks in between, while others are natural-born grazers.

Struggling with food—the neophobic response

You may find that your child is neophobic, but this doesn't mean a trip to the doctor, just an in-built fear of new foods and new things in general. Essentially it's a survival technique, and understanding it will help to explain why your child can seemingly switch from a happy-go-lucky "I'll taste anything" babe to an "If you think I'm eating that you're nuts" toddler. The neophobic response kicks in at around the age your child learns to crawl and walk and is beginning to explore away from the watchful eyes of adults. Previously your child will have happily put anything into their mouths. Now, however, they will become increasingly skeptical and extremely cautious when they encounter foods they don't recognize, either flatly refusing or spitting out alien substances. One way to introduce new foods is to mix them in with foods you know they like. It's important not to give up, since a more varied diet at this stage should mean your child is less picky later.

Brain food

Children's food intake, at this age, is like a yo-yo. Your child might eat a continent-sized lunch, but an itsy-bitsy-teeny-weeny dinner. Just go with the flow. As Elizabeth Morse says in *My Child Won't Eat*, "If a child grew at the same rate as in the first year, they would be 95 feet long and weigh 441,000 pounds by the age of ten." A toddler's appetite does lose momentum, but they will need a steady stream of food as their brain is dissecting and processing information. At this age, it's not surprising that two-thirds of their food is used by the brain. To keep their blood sugar up, small people need to eat and drink every two to three hours—even if it's just a snack.

A rough guide to a 2-year-old's daily intake

You don't need a meal planner for this stage, but here is a checklist so that you can make sure your child is getting a good mix of the food groups below.

3–4 servings of fruit and veg

(an apple, a peach, broccoli florets, lettuce, and tomatoes)

3–5 servings of carbohydrate

(a slice of bread, a serving of potatoes, a bowl of pasta)

3 servings of dairy food

(a fromage frais, yogurt, slices of cheese, a glass of warm milk)

1 serving of animal protein or
2 servings of vegetable protein

(1 egg, 1 peanut butter sandwich, a serving of fish, chicken or beef, tofu, pulses, nuts)

Avoiding food fights

Eating is one of life's great pleasures, so try to keep mealtimes breezy and fun. The minute you start force-feeding, bribing, or cajoling your child with food, mealtimes can become a power struggle. Though a child may learn that, "Yuck, I don't like it" can get them yummier alternatives, the challenge for you is to find out whether they are not eating simply because they're not feeling too well, they're teething, they don't like the taste or texture of the food, or because there are more exciting things to do.

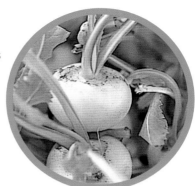

Here are some ways to avoid food stand-offs

One of the golden rules of getting your baby to eat is to eat with them

If you've eaten alone in a restaurant, you'll know it can be a disconcerting experience, so don't be surprised if your baby struggles to eat under your beady eye. If your baby sees you tucking in too, however, they'll be inspired to do the same.

Vary the venue. If you've reached a stand-off, simply transport them to somewhere different, like a picnic rug on the living-room floor or an outdoor space if you have one.

It's perfectly normal for your baby to love a food one week and loathe it the next

Just take it away and try it again later.

Make sure that the food is neither too hot nor too cold. Most babies love warm food because it's reminiscent of breast milk and easy to swallow. However, try to present them with slight variations in temperature, so you don't end up with a fussy toddler who won't eat cold food.

It's not unusual for an independent weaner to get annoyed when you try to feed them, particularly rejecting smooth purées in favor of foods they find easier to feed themselves with. Conversely don't be surprised if on off-days they are more than happy to be mommy's or daddy's little baby again and relish the comfort of being spoon-fed.

Avoid overloading your baby's plate because too much food can seem overwhelming

Instead, give your baby a small amount and give them loads of praise when it's gone down the hatch before spooning out more (for example, "Oh—you are a great eater. I wonder if you can eat some more").

Note Babies of this age are getting smarter and may realize that if they fuss enough and refuse to eat their main course they'll get an alternative, like yogurt or cookies. Keep desserts as an occasional treat. If they do get fussy, just remove the plate and don't offer anything else except maybe a piece of fruit or a slice of cheese until the next meal by which time they should be very hungry. While a child may assert their independence, they will never starve themselves.

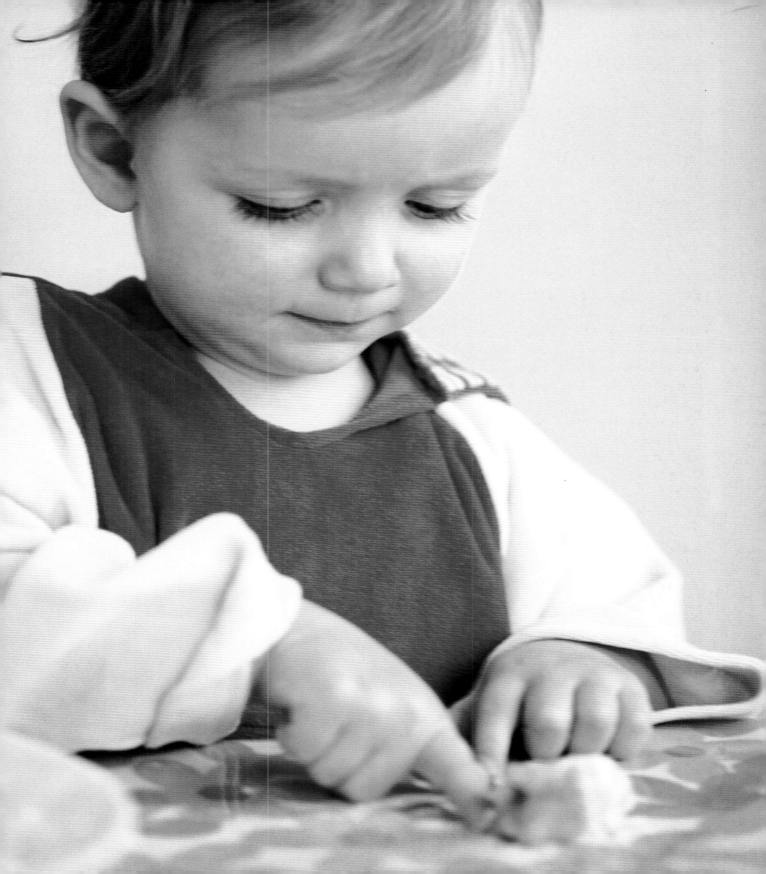

Breakfast to go

Breakfast can be a social time, even if it is a bit dine and dash. If you're a working parent most days you won't have time to create a fresh breakfast from scratch so a pantry full of homemade mueslis and bread variations is quick and easy. Here is a handful of recipes (don't forget the recipes in the earlier sections too) that take a few minutes to rustle up and provide your child with a morning's worth of good nutrition. Some of these ideas make excellent desserts or snacks too.

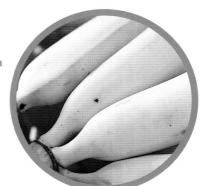

Banana Toast with Yogurt

Cooking in butter, for a minute, caramelizes the banana into a sticky delight. For this recipe you could also use raisin or fruit bread, pannetone, or just a plain wholemeal muffin.
Makes 1 serving

1 tablespoon unsalted butter
1 ripe banana
2 tablespoons maple syrup
Pinch of cinnamon

Sprinkling of finely chopped toasted almonds (if not allergic)
1 slice of raisin or fruit bread
Dollop of yogurt

Melt the butter in a nonstick skillet. Peel and diagonally slice the banana and fry for a minute or two. Add the maple syrup, a pinch of cinnamon, and mix in the almonds, if using.

Toast and butter the bread and cut into triangles or wedges. Spoon on the banana mixture and serve with yogurt and a dusting of cinnamon.

Groovy Granola

Make a big batch of this on a Sunday (you may want to double the recipe) and store in an airtight container. Involve your child in selecting what they want in their granola—they could name it too. This also makes a good topping for apple crumble or a healthy granola bar.
Makes 2–3 servings

1 tablespoon sunflower seeds
1 tablespoon pumpkin seeds
1 dessertspoon linseeds (flax seeds)
1/3 cup hazelnuts (omit if there is a nut allergy)

1 1/2 cups rolled oats
2 tablespoons sunflower oil
2 tablespoons organic honey
1/2 cup golden raisins or raisins

Preheat the oven to 350°F.

Grind up all the seeds (and nuts if using) roughly in a blender and combine with the oats on a baking sheet.

Melt the sunflower oil and honey together in a saucepan and pour this mixture into the baking sheet, making sure all the oat mixture gets a good coating.

Bake for about 30 minutes, stirring occasionally, until the mixture is golden. Remove from the oven and mix in the raisins. Store in an airtight container. Serve with milk or yogurt and fresh fruit.

Eggs: Scrambled or Bang Bang!

It's quick, it's nutritious, it's scramblers with hot, unsalted-buttered toast. Alternatively go for Bang Bang Eggs aka boiled egg—which sounds more fun and will remind them that they get to crack the top with a spoon. Serve with toast fingers. Eggs need to be hard boiled for babies and young children.

Makes 1 serving

1 egg   1 tablespoon whole milk
½ teaspoon olive oil

Heat a small saucepan on the stove. Beat together all the ingredients in a bowl, then pour into the pan. Stir continuously until the mixture is just moist (but not dry). Serve on toast or rolled in a fresh soft tortilla.

For extra nutrition and variety, you can add a number of ingredients to the mixture, like grated cheese, flaked tuna fish (canned in oil or water, not brine), tomatoes, or finely chopped peppers.

If you want Bang Bang Eggs, hardboil the egg for 8–10 minutes.

Purple Oatmeal

Hard to compete with the free gizmos and promotions of the commercial cereals—and some are great for kids, especially served with fresh fruit for sweetness and variety, but others are high in refined sugar, which will give your child a quick burst of energy that'll make them crash and burn.

Compared to packaged cereals, homemade oatmeal may seem dull, dull, dull, so here's a recipe that gets away from the usual brown mush—and is a hit with kids and adults alike. And yes, it really is bright purple!

Makes 1 serving

⅓ cup rolled oats   ⅓ cup fresh or frozen
½ cup milk   summer fruits
1 teaspoon sunflower kernals   (blackcurrants, redcurrants,
  (whole or ground)   cherries, raspberries,
1 teaspoon pumpkin kernals   strawberries, blackberries)
  (whole or ground)   1 teaspoon honey

Combine all the ingredients in a medium saucepan and bring to a boil. Reduce the heat and simmer for 5–8 minutes, until the oats are soft, and serve as is or with yogurt.

To freeze your own summer fruits, remove all stalks and pits, rinse in a colander, and drain. Spread the fruits on a large baking sheet and freeze for 1–2 hours. Bag up into small freezer bags, date, and label. If you bag up soft fruits without pre-freezing, you will end up with a solid clump; this method helps to keep them loose.

Vegetables: the art of disguise

This can be a tricky age when it comes to eating vegetables and I often hear parents lamenting that their children won't eat greens. If your child is a late starter, I recommend the art of disguise as a short-term fix, but in the long term you'll need to get them acquainted. One way is to offer your child a little raw or cooked vegetable with each meal, so they can feel, see, and smell them. While you're hiding vegetables in, under, or around foods that you know your child will eat, also put out new foods to introduce them to. Instead of expecting them to try foods out of the blue, present the food a dozen times over a period of weeks. Just as curiosity got the cat, your tot will eventually try them.

Children are notoriously picky. For 2-year-olds their version of a gastronomic delight is buttered toast, while broccoli can be an alien life form. Get your toddler to help you prepare the food. They can wash vegetables, add chopped vegetables to dishes, stir and play "tester"—it all helps to break down the barriers.

Many children are averse to fresh produce being introduced at this stage, particularly if they have been weaned on commercial baby food, which is generally monotextured and bland. If this is the case, you may need to rewean your toddler. Take them back a step to more mashed foods, then try finely diced foods and finally whole foods. Children are also more likely to accept—and taste—new foods that are similar to foods they know. If, for example, they like peaches, nectarines aren't a big deviation. Or, if they like a meat burger, they'll like a chicken burger or a veggie burger.

Another way is to serve their favorite dish with a few variations (scrambled eggs with smoked salmon, mushrooms, cheese). And, of course, anything can be disguised when it's squashed between two bits of bread or rolled up in a tortilla.

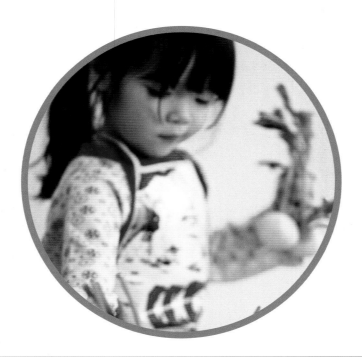

Secret Agent Sauce aka Hidden Vegetable Sauce

Makes 2–4 servings

FOR THE BASIC SAUCE
2 tablespoons red onion
1 teaspoon olive oil
¼ cup carrot
¼ cup sweet potato
¾ ounce fresh medium beet or 1 cube beet purée (see page 66)
2–3 tablespoons water
¼ cup red pepper

1 small ripe tomato
¼ cup broccoli
¼ cup zucchini
¼ cup spinach
3–4 button mushrooms
1 garlic clove
1–2 tablespoons whole milk
1 teaspoon Worcestershire sauce
Freshly ground black pepper

Finely chop the onion and gently cook with the olive oil in a small saucepan. Wash, peel, and finely chop the carrot and sweet potato (if using fresh beet, finely peel, chop, and add here) and add to the onion, cook for a further 3 minutes then add the water and gently simmer.

Wash and finely chop the red pepper, tomato, broccoli, zucchini, spinach, mushrooms, and garlic and add with the milk. Simmer for a further 4 minutes. If using beet purée, stir through a little at a time to color the sauce to the desired red.

Purée with a hand blender to the appropriate texture for your child. Season with Worcestershire sauce and pepper to taste.

Quick sauce method: if you have a younger child who is weaning or about to and you have frozen cubes of purée, simply sweat the onion with the olive oil and add in a cube of the various purées. Heat until defrosted. Wash and finely chop the tomato and red pepper and stir in with the milk (and, if needed, additional water). Blend as before.

Serve on pasta, adding crème fraîche, mascarpone cheese, or grated hard cheese to make it creamy and to add protein, or use instead of ketchup.

Mighty Meaty Pasta Sauce

A meat pasta sauce hides a multitude of vegetable sins, but made this way it also provides iron coupled with vitamin-rich vegetables. Just as with the Secret Agent Sauce, feel free to chop and change the hidden vegetables to what's in season or whatever you know you'll get away with hiding—such as spinach in place of peas.

Makes 1 serving

1 teaspoon olive oil
½ medium onion
1 garlic clove
2–3 ounces lean mince (beef, lamb, chicken, turkey)
¼ red pepper
3–4 button mushrooms
1 dessertspoon fresh or frozen peas
¼ cup carrot (or 1 cube carrot purée, see page 60)

¼ cup sweet potato (or 1 cube sweet potato purée, see page 60)
1 medium tomato (or 1 canned plum tomato)
½ teaspoon tomato purée
1 tablespoon water or stock (see page 118)
¼ teaspoon oregano
1 tablespoon fresh parsley

Heat the oil in a nonstick skillet. Dice, peel, and finely chop the onion and crush the garlic and gently cook in the oil until the onion starts to soften. Increase the heat slightly, add the ground meat and keep stirring until the meat is cooked and just begins to brown, then reduce the heat to low.

Wash, peel, and finely chop the other vegetables and add to the mixture (grate the carrot and sweet potato to speed up cooking time along with the remaining ingredients). Gently simmer until all the vegetables are soft, then beat with a hand blender to a fairly smooth sauce.

Serve over a bed of spaghetti, on top of freshly cooked mashed or baked potatoes topped with cheese, or allow to cool and freeze until needed.

Vegetable ice creams

You probably think I'm having a laugh if I imagine any of you are going near these. But if I told you, or more importantly a child who doesn't like vegetables, that I had some delicious purple ice cream or an orange frozen yogurt, you wouldn't be surprised to find children are quite willing to try my Frankenstein creations. And, just to encourage you, not one of the groups of parents I tried these on was able to tell me what was in Cabbage or Brussels Sprout Ice Cream. So don't be scared and remember you're not creating a monster but a masterpiece.

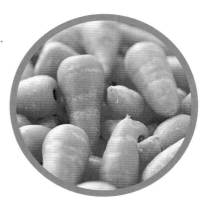

Frozen Yogurt

Parsnip and Pear Frozen Yogurt or White Ice Cream

1 cup parsnip	1 cup whole natural yogurt
¾ cup very ripe pear	

Wash and peel the parsnip, removing the tough center core and grate or very finely chop. Wash, peel, core, and grate the pear. Put the parsnip and the pear in a saucepan with just enough boiling water to cover, reduce the heat, and simmer for 10–15 minutes until the largest piece of parsnip is soft.

Blend in the chopping attachment of a hand blender until smooth, pour into a container, and cover. Set aside to cool, then chill in the refrigerator.

Stir 1½ cups of the parsnip and pear purée into the yogurt. Churn in an ice cream maker until thick, then scoop individual portions into lidded, freezer-proof containers. Freeze until required.

Note All recipes require an ice cream maker (see manufacturer's instructions for use).
Homemade ice cream can be stored for up to 3 months in a standard domestic freezer.

Carrot and Orange Frozen Yogurt or Orange Ice Cream

If your child likes the sharpness of citrus, replace a little of the orange juice with fresh lemon juice to make it super zingy.

1¼ cups carrot	1 cup whole natural yogurt
1 cup freshly squeezed orange juice	

Wash and peel the carrots and grate or very finely chop. Stir the carrot into the orange juice and bring to a boil in a medium saucepan. Reduce the heat and simmer for 10–15 minutes until the largest piece of carrot is soft and the juice has reduced in volume by about one-third.

Beat in the chopping attachment of a hand blender until smooth, pour into a container, and cover. Set aside to cool, then chill in the refrigerator.

Stir 1½ cups of the carrot and orange purée into the yogurt. Churn in an ice cream maker until thick, then scoop individual portions into lidded, freezer-proof containers. Freeze until required.

Ice Creams

Minty Pea Ice Cream

1–4 sprigs of fresh mint
1²⁄₃ cups frozen peas

½ cup whipping cream
½ cup whole milk

Wash the mint and tear or coarsely chop (vary the quantity to suit your child).

Bring to a boil just enough water to cover the mint and peas, add, then reduce to a simmer for 10 minutes until the peas are very soft. Beat in the chopping attachment of a hand blender, adding the water the peas were cooked in to make a glossy, smooth purée.

Pour into a container and cover. Set aside to cool, then chill in the refrigerator. Stir 1½ cups of the minty pea purée into the cream and milk. Churn in an ice cream maker until thick, then scoop individual portions into lidded, freezer-proof containers. Freeze until required.

Purple or Creamy Green Ice Cream

Red cabbage gives this a lovely natural purple color and the apple and raisins soften the bitterness. Vary the amount of cinnamon to suit your child. If your child takes to this, why not get ambitious and try Brussels sprouts?

¾ cup red cabbage or
  8 Brussels sprouts
⅓ cup dessert apple
2 tablespoons golden raisins

1 tablespoon butter
½ teaspoon cinnamon
½ cup whipping cream
½ cup whole milk

Wash and finely shred the cabbage. Wash, peel, core, and grate the apple and rinse the raisins. Melt the butter in a medium saucepan, reduce the heat, then stir in the cabbage, apple, sultanas, and cinnamon. Cook for 2–3 minutes, stirring frequently to avoid burning. Add 2–4 tablespoons of water, bring to a boil, then immediately reduce to a gentle simmer for 10 minutes. Check that the largest piece of cabbage is soft. Blend, using the chopping attachment of a hand blender to make a glossy, very smooth purée.

Pour into a container and cover. Set aside to cool, then chill in the refrigerator. Stir the cabbage purée into the cream and milk. Churn in an ice cream maker until thick, then scoop individual portions into lidded, freezer-proof containers. Freeze until required.

Green Ice Cream

This recipe is the most savory tasting of these recipes—think of a light frozen herb butter rather than an ice cream. Serve on its own or with hot broiled meat, poultry, or fish and mashed potato. It will melt to give a savory creamy sauce.

¾ cup broccoli
½ cup leeks
4–5 basil leaves

½ cup whole milk
1 egg yolk
½ cup whipping cream

Wash and trim the stalks of the broccoli and leeks, then finely chop. Rinse the basil leaves. Bring all except 1 tablespoon of the milk to a boil, then add the broccoli, leek, and basil. Return to the boil, then simmer for 10–12 minutes until the largest piece is soft. Push the mix through a strainer, reserving the cooking milk, and purée the vegetables in the chopping attachment of a hand blender until glossy, and very smooth, adding a little of the boiled milk as needed.

Beat the egg yolk with the remaining milk, then pour into the saucepan with the rest of the boiled milk. Cook for 4–5 minutes over a gentle heat, stirring continuously until it thickens slightly, but don't let it boil since this will cause the mixture to separate (if your child has an egg allergy, the recipe will work without the egg custard). Put the puréed vegetable mixture, milk, and egg in lidded containers and set aside to cool, then chill in the refrigerator.

Combine 1 cup of the broccoli purée with the egg custard and cream. Churn in an ice cream maker until thick, then scoop individual portions into lidded, freezer-proof containers. Freeze until required.

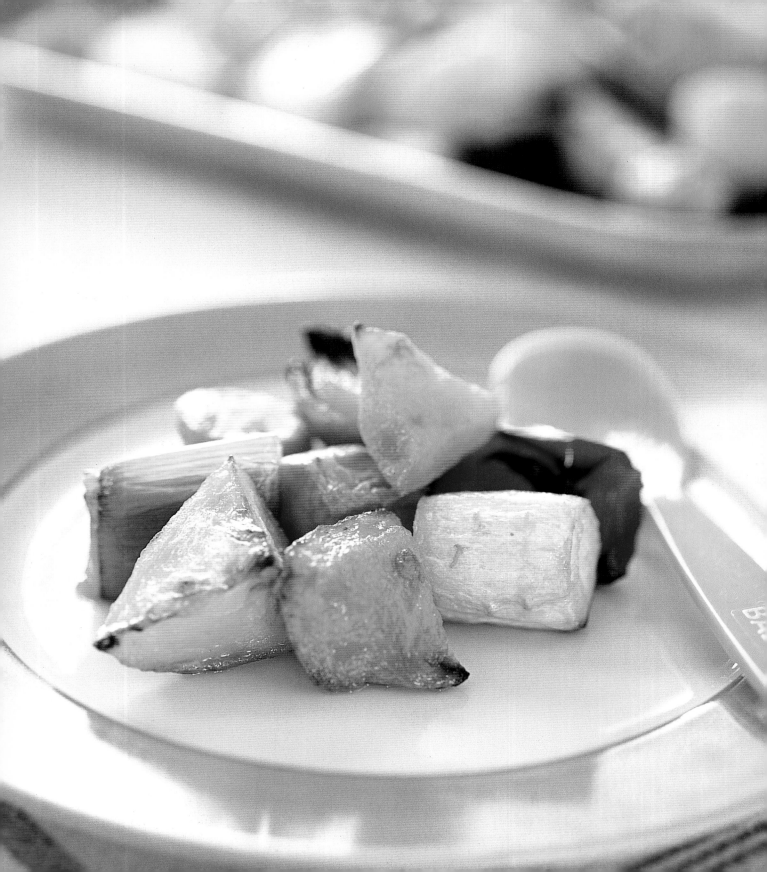

Jazz 'em up

If you are having trouble getting your little one to eat vegetables and your cunning disguises are as much use as a newspaper with eyeholes cut out, then go the other way and make the vegetables the exciting part of their meal. If all else fails, get them to help you wash, peel, and chop the vegetables because, as you know, it's harder to turn your nose up at something when you know the amount of effort that's been put in.

Roast Them All

The roast potato is familiar to all of us, but why stop there? This recipe is a quick and easy way to prepare lots of vegetables at once—the slow roast gives you the time to do other things while filling the kitchen with delicious aromas.
Makes 1–4 servings (depending on how many vegetables you prepare)

3–4 tablespoons olive oil
2 garlic cloves crushed
  (optional)
2 sprigs of fresh rosemary
  (optional)

A selection of the following:
1 carrot
1/2 cup pumpkin/squash (e.g.
  butternut squash or red kuri)
1 medium potato

1 sweet potato
1 parsnip
1 beetroot
1–2 baby leeks
2–3 shallots
1/2 red or green pepper
1/2 cup yam

Preheat the oven to 350ºF .

Heat the olive oil in a large roasting pan with the garlic and rosemary, if using.

Wash, peel, and chop the selection of vegetables roughly into 3/4 inch cubes.

When the oven is ready, toss the medley of vegetables in the oil and roast for 30–40 minutes, turning them a couple of times. Cook until crispy and browning on the outside, soft on the inside. Once cooked, simply reduce the heat to 275ºF and cook slowly for up to 40 minutes to enhance the flavor.

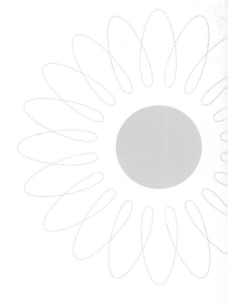

Tempura Vegetables

Tempura vegetables are fried, so they should not be eaten at every meal, but they make a quick, special treat when friends are visiting or if you are trying to get a child's interest back into the world of vegetables. Just like a box of chocolates, part of the fun of tempura is not knowing what's inside—the cheese chunks will be a gooey surprise.
Makes 2 servings (not suitable for freezing)

A selection of the following:	1 tablespoon cornstarch
½ carrot	½ teaspoon olive oil
4 sugarsnap peas	1 tablespoon water
4 button mushrooms	1 egg white (for an idea of
2 baby corn	what to do with the yolk see
4 small florets broccoli	Cheesy Footballs recipe,
½ zucchini	page 162)
4 chunks of pineapple	
4 chunks of cheese	
1 cup sunflower oil	

Prepare the vegetables. Thinly slice the carrot and halve the sugarsnap peas, mushrooms, and baby corn. Cut the zucchini into chunks.

Fill a wok or deep skillet 1¼–1½ inches deep with oil (note: this recipe does not work with olive oil because olive oil will not get hot enough).

Mix the cornstarch with the olive oil and water. Beat the egg white until stiff and fold into the cornstarch mixture. Pour the chopped ingredients into the fluffy batter.

Heat the oil and deep fry the chunks in batches, 4–5 at a time. The batter will swell and crispen. Turn once to make sure the tempura are golden on each side and use a slotted spoon to remove. Lay the pieces on a couple of sheets of paper towel to soak up the excess oil. Repeat until finished.

Serve immediately.

Stir Fry

This oriental method of cooking is often a hit with kids since it combines the crunch of raw food with the comfort of hot food. Typically sesame or peanut oils are used; however both are known to be a higher allergy risk, so if in any doubt stick to olive oil (as this recipe suggests).
Makes 1–2 servings

Select a colorful combination from the following:	¼ cup beansprouts or alfalfa
½ carrot	¼ cup water chestnuts (canned)
½ stick of celery	¼ cup bamboo shoots (canned)
½ zucchini	¼ cup pak choi
2 green onions	
2–3 mushrooms	
4–5 snow peas	1–2 tablespoons olive oil
4–5 string beans	1 garlic clove, crushed (optional)
½ cup spinach leaves	1 tablespoon low-salt soy sauce
¼ cup cabbage	Juice of ¼ lime
2–3 baby corn	
3–4 small broccoli florets	
¼ red, green, or yellow pepper	

Wash, peel and slice your selection of ingredients into bite-sized pieces.

Heat the oil in a nonstick wok (or large nonstick skillet) with the crushed garlic, if using. Put the chopped ingredients into the pan and stir frequently to coat and heat through. Some children like the taste of the slightly browned bits, so vary the cooking time to suit your child. Toss in the soy and lime juice, then serve.

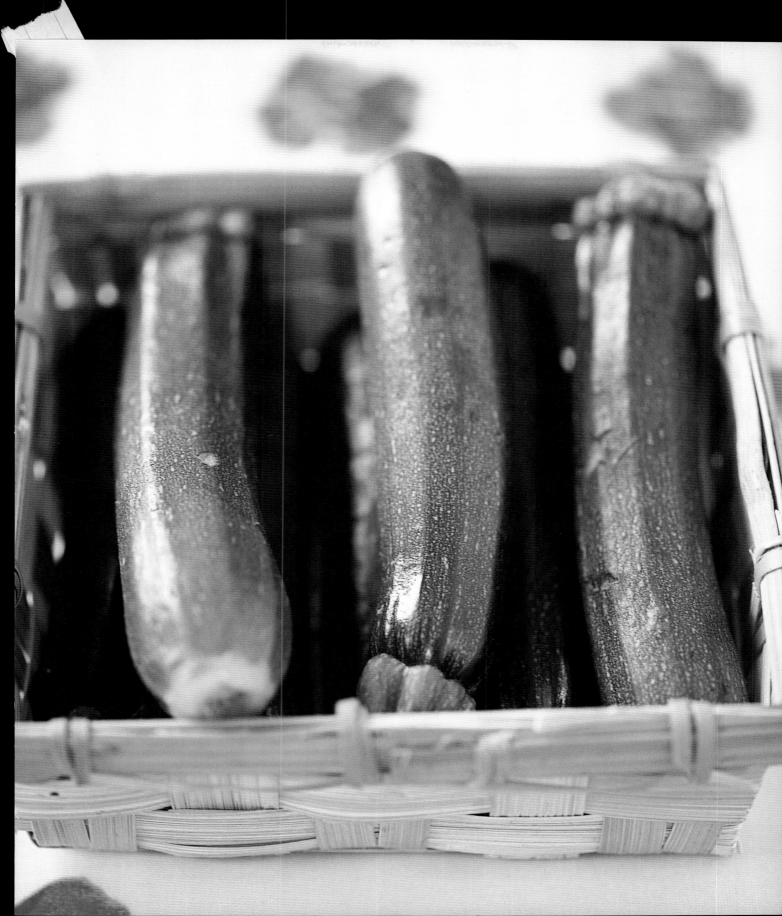

Keeping it simple

While some children like mixed-up food, others like to see what they're eating. They like their food b[...]

Serving food in compartments means they'll get an array of appetizing foods from which they can r[...]

you're using saucepans, you could go crazy, so try using a steamer with dividing walls, which will he[...] k small

amounts separated at the same time, including fish, meat, and rice. Raw food can be harder to digest so another

option is to part-steam the vegetables then serve warm or cold.

Simple Steamers

¼ **pound chicken fillet**	**1 tablespoon sweetcorn**
⅓ **cup broccoli**	**1 small carrot**

Cut the chicken into small strips. Wash, then cut or break the broccoli into small florets, slice off the corn from a cob (or use unsweetened corn canned in water not brine). Wash, peel, and slice the carrot into fine sticks.

Using the dividers, steam the ingredients separately and serve on a plate with divisions or a large plate with plenty of space in between.

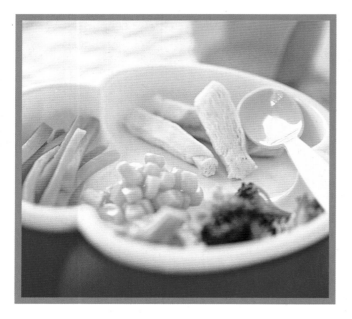

Vegetable Pick 'n' Mix

Most adults like a big bowl of salad with everything mixed but some children find this too messy. Try keeping all the vegetables separate so your child can pick 'n' mix. If one particular vegetable is left, you can work out why your child doesn't like mixed salad.

Children may also take to separated salads since the crunch of some foods like cabbage can make them more appealing raw than cooked.

Remember to select a variety of colors as a quick way to balance nutrition.

Select a colorful combination from the following:
Red and yellow peppers
Cabbage
Cherry tomatoes
Sweet potato
Carrot
Cauliflower
Snow peas
Celery
Cucumber
Avocado

Making mealtime a learning time

Food and eating can become boring compared to toys, videos, and TV programs. Try looking at mealtimes as a learning time. Clear the table of toys and distractions and set it for both of you. Turn off the TV or radio and treat it as a special "us" time.

Rather than creating artistic masterpieces think creatively about themes relating to what they're into at the moment and what they're learning about at playgroup, on TV, or in their favorite book. Think of eating as part of the learning rather than the main focus of mealtime. Here are a few ideas to get you started.

Learning to count
OK, this is very easy. You could line the food up like a multicolored abacus (1 slice of zucchini, 2 slices of carrot, 3 pieces of yellow pepper, 4 cherry tomatoes, 5 grapes). Or line up 1 homemade chicken/fish/veggie strip, 2 boiled potatoes, 3 baby carrots, 4 string beans. They can subtract them by eating them. And then how many are left?

Colors
On a large plate, place a selection of different-colored foods and ask, "What color are the peas?" If they get it right, they can eat them and so on.

Face-off
Almost any meal can be turned into a face. This is quick and easy to do. For example, with a salad, just halve 2 yellow cherry tomatoes for eyes, use raisins as eyeballs, add a nose with a sausage; use a wedge of red pepper for a mouth and sliced hard-boiled-egg moon shapes for ears. Create hair from cooked pasta in pesto or mashed potato. It's even easier with fruit. Try a couple of grapes for eyes, half a banana for a nose, an apple wedge for a mouth, raisins for the hair, and a couple of tangerine wedges for the ears.

Clock-face
Place peas or sliced cooked or raw carrots (or zucchini, potatoes, or whatever you like) around the rim of a plate. Make the clock hands from carrots, cheese, red or green pepper, or celery cut lengthwise. Create the "centerpiece" from a homemade burger, egg, or a pile of tuna, ham, or other source of protein. Then your child can eat every "number" the hands point to!

Giant's dinner or witch's playground
This one just involves creating a "landscape" from food. For example, make a forest from broccoli "trees," towers of carrots (just stand them on end), mountains of mash, bolder cherry tomatoes… you've got it in one.

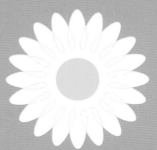

Healthy fast food

Fast food is not necessarily junk food. No doubt you'll have decided you will never feed your child burgers or chicken nuggets. Don't do it. Before you set a hard rod for your back, don't forget that banning foods is a surefire way to make them more attractive to a belligerent toddler. Right now, "junk foods" are a hot potato in the food industry, but the truth is snacks and food in a flash can be healthy. Yes, even burgers and chicken nuggets.

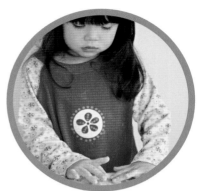

Home Burgers (Classic, Salmon, and Vegetable)

A chameleon of a recipe: fish, meat, or poultry, smooth or chunky to suit your child's fancy. Keep it simple with the basic recipe, or select from the optional extras to add in a few hidden vegetables.
Makes 10 small burgers

BASIC RECIPE
¾ pound salmon or trout fillet, skinned and chopped into ¼ inch cubes
or
¾ pound ground beef, lamb, pork, turkey, or chicken or chopped into ¼ inch cubes
½ medium onion
¾ cup oats
1 medium egg
1 tablespoon flour (yellow corn or plain wheat)
1 tablespoon olive oil

OPTIONAL EXTRAS
1 tablespoon finely chopped, fresh, herbs (e.g. cilantro, tarragon, basil, mint, oregano, or parsley)
Pinch of mild spice, e.g. paprika, cumin, turmeric
1 tablespoon shredded spinach
1 garlic clove, crushed
1 tablespoon chopped red or yellow pepper
1 tablespoon finely chopped mushrooms
(Additional beaten egg may be needed to bind the drier ingredients)

In a large mixing bowl, combine the fish or meat with the onion, oats, and selection (if any) from the optional list. Beat the egg and stir into the mix. For a smooth-textured burger, mix using a hand blender to make a thick, smooth paste.

To form the patties, flour the inside of a mug, drop in a tablespoon of burger mixture and sprinkle in a little more flour. Firmly squash down the mixture using the blunt end of a rolling pin or back of a spoon. Run a rounded-end knife around the sides of the mix, invert the mug, and a formed pattie will drop out. Repeat for the rest of the mixture.

Heat a little olive oil in a nonstick skillet. Place the burgers in the oil and cook for about 5 minutes on each side until golden brown.

Serve in a warmed pita pocket or roll with salad or steamed vegetables. Delicious with Secret Agent Sauce (see page 147).

Tip If your child prefers the basic recipe smooth and you like the chunkier version, take out a couple of tablespoons to blend, then add your favorite combinations to the remaining mixture.

Fast food, not junk food

The thing is, "junk" fast foods are often made from junk ingredients, but when you make your own at home, you know exactly what's in them. Take pizza, for example, which gets a bad press because the typical take-out is made with a base of refined white flour, bound with hydrogenated oils, lathered with cheap oily cheese, processed meats, barely fresh vegetables, and often coated with salt. When you make it yourself, you can make a far healthier version.

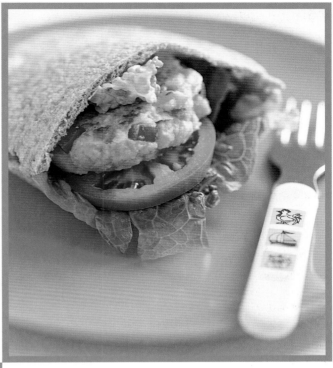

Regular snacking

Toddlers needs to eat every 2–3 hours. Snacks are therefore a part of their dietary landscape. What you need to give them are snacks with a good GI (glycemic index) rating (50 or below) to keep their little AA-sized batteries lasting longer. Choosing the wrong food to satisfy hunger is a primary cause of childhood obesity, so instead of instant-rush potato chips, soda, and candy, your child needs foods to help supply their brain with a steady stream of glucose and to prevent them from having temper tantrums that put prima donnas to shame.

Keep "good" snacks (e.g. boxes of raisins, carrot batons, apple slices, or satsuma segments) to hand, with a selection tucked in your stroller bag or car glove compartment, so you're not tempted to rush into a grocery store and buy one of the glinting fat/sugar/salt-laden bags on offer.

Pizza

A hit with all the family, there are limitless variations of what to put on a pizza—below are just a few suggestions. You can include the chosen topping in with the basic tomato sauce (and blending to a smoother paste) or sprinkle on top before adding the cheese so that they're easy to see.
Makes 3–4 servings (1 large or 4 individual pizzas)

FOR THE BASE
Double the quantities of No-salt Breadsticks dough (see page 126) and add:
2 tablespoons whole or chopped sunflower kernals and pumpkin kernals

1 tablespoon olive oil to grease a baking tray

FOR THE BASIC TOPPING SAUCE
1 tablespoon olive oil
1 cup onions
1–2 garlic cloves
1 cup fresh or tinned tomatoes
1 teaspoon chopped capers or olives (optional)
1 teaspoon fresh or 1/2 teaspoon dried mixed herbs
1/2 teaspoon vinegar or Worcestershire sauce
Freshly ground black pepper

TO SPRINKLE ON TOP OR BLEND IN WITH THE TOPPING SAUCE
SELECT FROM
1/2 cup zucchini
1/2 cup mushrooms
1/2 cup red or green pepper

TO FINISH
2/3 cup hard cheese

Preheat the oven to 425°F. Make the dough, adding the kernals before the water. Set aside to allow to rise.

To make the topping, heat the oil in a medium saucepan. Peel and chop the onions, crush the garlic and cook until soft. Chop the tomatoes and add with the capers or olives (if using), herbs, vinegar, or Worcestershire sauce and black pepper. Stir well and bring to a simmer.

Chop your selected topping ingredients and if you want a smooth sauce, add to the tomato mixture and blend.

Flour a clean work surface and either stretch or roll out the dough to the size of your baking sheet. Oil the baking sheet and put the dough on to the sheet, stretching to fit as needed.

Spread the sauce on the base, sprinkle with the topping if not blended in the sauce (encourage your child to do this to make it their handiwork), and grate the cheese on top.

Bake for 25–30 minutes until the dough edges sound hollow when you tap them and the cheese begins to brown.

Serve, or cool and freeze. Delicious hot or cold.

Fish Cakes

Unlike burgers, a good fish cake should be a meal in itself, with a nice balance of fish, potato, and vegetable. You can vary this recipe by replacing the fish with a lean minced meat.
Makes 8 fish cakes

1/2 cup potato or sweet potato
1/4 cup carrot
1/4 cup leek
1/4 cup baby sweetcorn
1/4 cup broccoli or peas
2 ounces skinless white fish

A little chopped dill (optional)
1/2 beaten egg
2/3 cup breadcrumbs
1–2 teaspoons olive oil
A little all-purpose flour

Wash, peel, and chop the potato and carrot. Steam for 5 minutes.

Finely slice the leek, baby sweetcorn, broccoli (or peas), add to the potatoes and carrot and steam for a further 5 minutes.

Check the fish for bones and finely chop. Add to the steamer with the dill, if using, and cook for 5 more minutes.

Meanwhile, beat the egg. Either mash or blend the vegetable and fish mixture depending on how coarse or smooth your child prefers it, adding in the egg.

Heat the olive oil in a skillet. Flour your hands then scoop a tablespoon-size dollop of the mixture and form a patty (the mixture will be quite moist), then drop into the breadcrumbs to coat. Fry on each side for 3–4 minutes until golden.

Meat Skewer Kebabs

Makes 3–4 skewers

¼ pound beef, lamb or turkey

8 button mushrooms

Red, yellow, or orange pepper

½ cup broccoli florets or a few mangetout

1 zucchini

¼ cup fresh or canned (in natural juice) pineapple or fresh mango

1–2 tablespoons olive oil

Preheat the broiler. Rinse and chop the meat, vegetables, and fruit to roughly ¾ inch cubes. Thread on to skewers making sure you have a bright combination of colors.

Brush with olive oil and broil for 6–7 minutes on each side until the meat is golden brown and cooked through.

Serve in pita breads with salad or with steamed vegetables.

Note Never give a young child a skewer—use a fork to slide the kebab off the skewer before serving.

Homemade Oven Fries

Russet, Burbank, and Kennebec are all great varieties for homemade oven fries. This method is part-boil, part-roast, which lowers the saturated fat content and avoids using a vat of hot oil.

Makes 1–2 servings

1 large potato

1 tablespoon sunflower oil

Preheat the oven to 400°F. Grease a non-stick baking sheet with half the oil and heat in the oven. Bring a pan of water to a boil while you wash and peel the potato and cut into chunky fries. Part-cook the fries in water by simmering for 3 minutes. Drain and dry off with paper towels. Place the fries on the baking sheet and drizzle with the remaining oil, making sure they are coated. Bake for 15 minutes, until golden and crispy, turning once, halfway through. Transfer to a plate and allow to cool before serving.

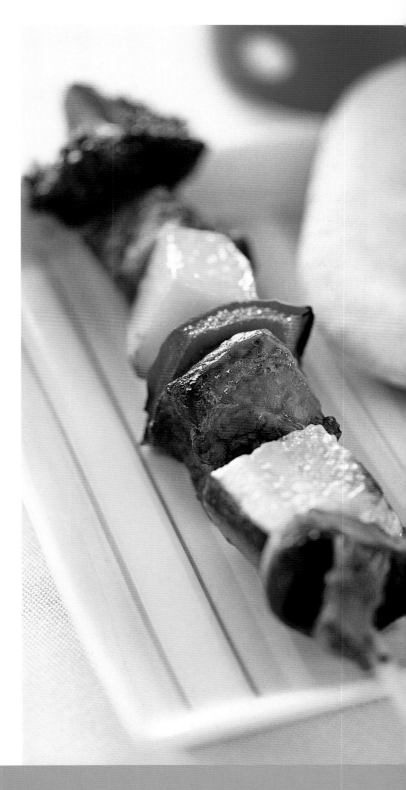

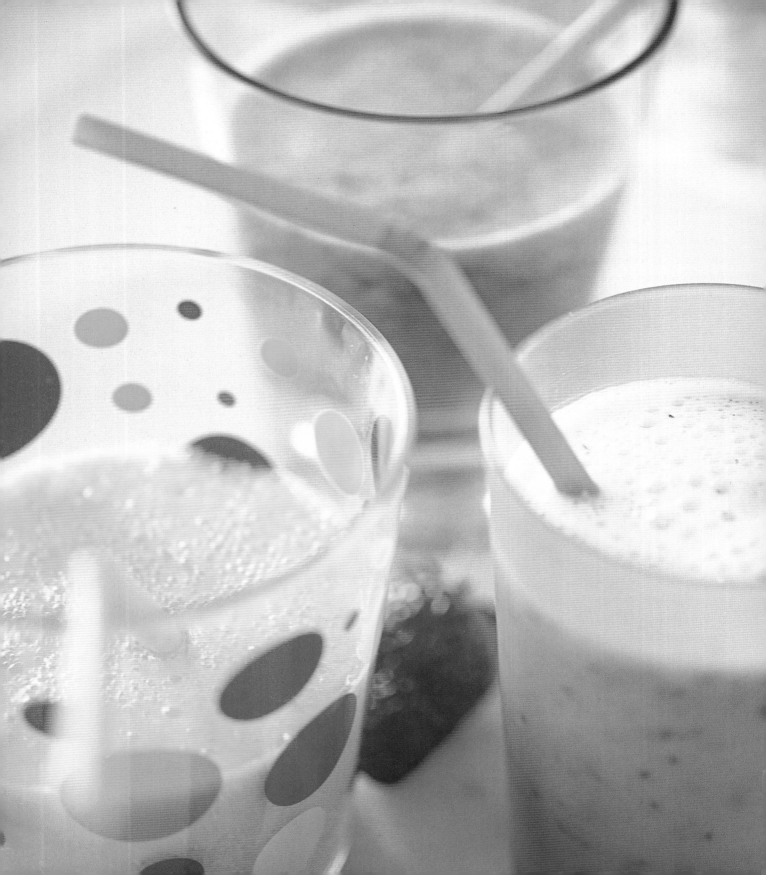

Drinks

You may know 5 pieces of fruit a day is the aim. However your toddler may not be so wise. Drinks are a great way to sneak a mix of fruit into their diets. Here are 4 fruity drinks to tempt your little ones.

Apple and Mint Lassi

Lassi originates from India, so it's deliciously refreshing on a hot day with the added benefit of being packed with calcium and vitamin D. The basic idea is fruit and yogurt and works well with most fruit. Use organic live yogurt. If your child doesn't like or can't have dairy, try a soybased yogurt.
Makes 1 tall drink

1/2 apple	1 cup iced water (or water
2–3 sprigs of fresh mint	and ice)
3 tablespoons natural yogurt	

Wash and core the apple (no need to peel). Combine all the ingredients in a blender and blend until smooth.

Serve immediately with a sprig of mint to garnish.

Strawberry Smoothie

The base of the smoothie is banana with a selection of fruit and some juice to keep it liquid. Smoothies are best chilled and work as well with frozen fruit. The variations are endless, but here's a simple one to get you started.
Makes 1 tall drink

1 medium banana	1 cup apple juice
1/3 cup strawberries (fresh or frozen)	

Combine all the ingredients in a blender and blend until smooth. If using fresh strawberries, include a few ice cubes to cool the drink.

Peach Melba Milkshake

Milkshakes may sound old-fashioned in this brave new world of smoothies, but made with fresh fruit, they are fab.
Makes 1 tall drink

1 peach	1 cup cow's milk, goat's milk
4–5 raspberries (fresh or frozen)	or soya milk

Peel the peach and remove the pit. Combine all the ingredients in a blender and blend until smooth. Serve immediately.

For a thick shake or a summer treat, replace 1/4 cup of milk with a scoop of ice cream.

Tropical Sunshine

The base of these is fruit and I can't think of a combination that would not work—it's a great way to enjoy seasonal fruits as well as a tropical treat even in winter.
Makes 1 tall drink

1/4 cup fresh mango	1 cup grapefruit or orange
1/4 cup fresh pineapple	juice

Combine all the ingredients in a blender and blend until smooth. Serve immediately

Some children (and adults) find grapefruit juice too bitter, so replace with orange juice, if preferred.

Snacks

Everybody from Scooby Doo to Homer Simpson likes a snack. Your little ones are no exception. With the amount of running around and growing taking place, it's important to keep energy levels balanced by storing some treats and having some handy recipes for when they come roaring into the kitchen.

Cheesy Footballs

Makes about 30
(these will freeze or keep in an airtight tin for up to a week)

1/4 stick butter or margarine, chilled
3/4 cup whole-wheat plain flour
1/2 cup cheddar cheese
Pinch of mustard (optional)
1 egg yolk (to use the egg

white, see Tempura Vegetables on page 152)
TO MAKE COLORED BALLS
1 teaspoon finely chopped or puréed red pepper or spinach
2–3 teaspoons milk if needed

Grate the butter into the flour and rub in until the mixture resembles breadcrumbs. Grate the cheese, stir into the flour and butter, and add the mustard, if using. Add the egg yolk and draw the mixture together to form a dough. If you are making colored balls, divide the dough and mix in the chopped or puréed pepper or spinach into half of the dough (adding the extra milk only if needed).

Put the dough in a plastic bag and chill for about 30 minutes. Meanwhile preheat the oven to 400°F. Lightly grease several baking sheets with a little olive oil or butter.

Lightly flour your hands, pull off a teaspoonful of dough, and roll into a ball. Place on the baking sheet and repeat using all the dough. Bake for 20 minutes until lightly golden. Transfer to a wire rack and allow to cool before serving.

Tip The dough can also be rolled out and shaped using a cookie cutter to any shape and become a savory version of Funny Face Biscuits on page 166.

Oat and Raisin Cookies

Makes 14 cookies
(these will freeze or keep in an airtight tin for up to a week)

1/4 stick butter
1/2 cup granulated sugar
1 egg, beaten
1/3 cup self-rising flour

2 cups rolled oats
1/2 cup raisins
1/2 teaspoon cinnamon

Preheat the oven to 350°F. Lightly grease two nonstick baking sheets.

In a large mixing bowl, cream together the butter and sugar until light and fluffy.

Add the beaten egg gradually and beat until well combined. Sift the flour into the creamed mixture, add the oats, raisins, and cinnamon and mix well.

Place tablespoonfuls of the mixture well apart on the prepared baking sheets and flatten them slightly with the back of a spoon. Bake for 15 minutes.

Leave the cookies to cool slightly on the baking sheets, before transferring to a wire rack. Leave to cool completely before serving.

Speedy Savory Pancakes

Makes 1–2 servings

¼ cup whole milk	1 tablespoon finely chopped
3 tablespoons whole-wheat	vegetables (choose from
or white self-rising flour	broccoli, corn, peppers,
1 small egg	peas, tomato)
3 tablespoons medium hard	1 tablespoon butter
cheese	

In a small mixing bowl gradually add the milk to the flour to avoid lumps. Beat the egg and add half to the mixture.

Grate the cheese and stir through the mixture. Add the vegetables.

Heat the butter in a nonstick skillet. Pour a tablespoonful of the mixture into the pan; it should spread to about 2 inches. Repeat to form another 2–3 pancakes, leaving a little space between each. Cook until they start to set and bubbles begin to form (about 3 minutes), then turn and cook for a further 3 minutes until golden.

Stuffed Mushrooms

Makes 6 stuffed mushrooms
(not suitable for freezing)

6 large button mushrooms	3 tablespoons hard cheese,
A little olive oil	grated
1 tablespoon fresh	1 garlic clove, crushed
breadcrumbs	1 teaspoon chopped chives

Wash and dry the mushrooms and remove the stalks. Brush the head with olive oil and gently broil until they begin to brown and soften a little (but not collapse).

Combine the breadcrumbs, cheese, garlic, and chives in the chopping bowl of a hand blender and mix. Use a teaspoon to pack the stuffing mixture into each mushroom and grill until golden.

Real Fruit Tarts

These can also be jam tarts (look out for some excellent low-sugar, high-in-real-fruit jams from specialist organic shops). Remember pastry should remain cold until it goes into a hot oven, so make sure that the fat is chilled; or if you have time make the dough in advance, pop it in a plastic bag, and chill or even freeze until needed.

Makes about 20 tarts

FOR THE PASTRY	2 muffin tins
¼ stick butter or margarine	FOR THE FILLING
(very cold)	Approx. 1 cup fruit purée
1⅔ cups whole-wheat plain	simmered to drive off excess
flour	liquid, then cooled
4–6 tablespoons very cold	Pinch of spice, e.g. cinnamon
water	or ginger (optional)

Grate the butter or margarine into the flour and lightly rub in. Add the water a little at a time and use a round-ended knife or metal spoon to mix and form a dough ball. You will need to use your fingers toward the end. Wrap in a plastic bag and either chill for at least 30 minutes or freeze for use on another day.

Preheat the oven to 425°F.

Roll out the pastry and cut into disks using a 3¼ inch pastry cutter. Place in the muffin tins. Put 1–2 teaspoons of fruit purée mixed with the spice or 1 frozen cube of fruit purée in each hole. Bake for 15–20 minutes. Allow to cool on a wire rack.

Fun with food and party ideas

You've probably had a good old belly laugh at cookbooks suggesting that parents present their children with complicated food sculptures. Ah—if only you had the time to fashion hairbows out of zucchini. In theory, though, it's a good idea because around this time your toddler's imagination begins to kick in—and one way to convince your child to eat is to tap into their fantasy world.

One of the problems with creating Picasso-like works of art is that you could find your child loves them so much they won't want to eat them. Some creations, like faces or clocks, are quick and easy to prepare (see Making mealtime a learning time on page 155); however, sometimes just re-naming the dishes makes them instantly more palatable. It's not spaghetti—it's shoelaces, slippery worms, or witch's hair. It's not just fish pie, it's Pingu's lunch or Bob the Builder's dinner.

Another way to get them to eat is by tapping into their fantasy world. It's not broccoli, it's a tree. A pea becomes a bolder. Mash becomes a mountain. Suddenly, dinner is not just a pile of vegetables—it's a giant's feast. Noises are another way to get them to eat their meals. After each mouthful, they can be a jeep and go "beep, beep" or a sheep and go "baa." You can also get an array of decorated utensils to have fun with (like an airplane or digger spoon). These can also come to life in their fantasy world, and you may just find them helpful with a food that is proving difficult.

While it's one way to get your child's eye connecting to their stomach, you don't want to make this a habit as mealtimes could turn very sour if every meal isn't some new, exciting adventure. Remind them that enjoying good-quality food is itself one of life's great pleasures.

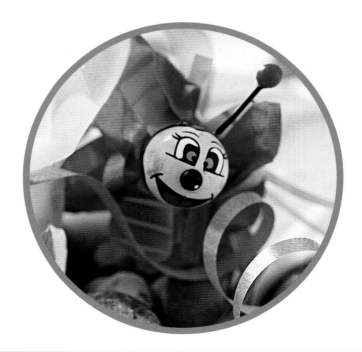

Dragon's Blood Soup

I have happy childhood memories of costume Halloween parties with a themed feast. Dragon's blood soup became a favorite not just on Halloween, but to warm up winter suppers too. To our neighbor's relief Mom couldn't find a dragon, so substituted tomatoes.

Makes 4–6 servings

2 pounds ripe tomatoes	2¼ cups milk or milk and
1 medium onion	stock (see page 118)
2 tablespoons butter,	½ teaspoon brown sugar
margarine or 1 tablespoon	1 small bay leaf
olive oil	1 tablespoon lemon juice
3 tablespoons cornflour	Freshly ground black pepper

Wash and finely chop the tomatoes and onion. Melt the butter or heat the oil and cook the tomatoes and onion until soft, then combine with a hand blender.

Blend the cornstarch with a little of the milk, making sure there are no lumps, then make up to 2¼ cups with the rest of the milk, stock if using, and sugar. Pour into the tomato purée, add the bay leaf and bring to a boil, stirring continuously. Simmer for 10 minutes, stirring occasionally. Toward the end of the 10 minutes, add the lemon juice and black pepper to taste. Remove the bay leaf.

Serve with Witch's Fingernails (see page 166). A sprinkling of grated cheese once served makes a special treat.

Other soup ideas

Dinosaur Swamp Soup
Use the Cheesy, Broccoli, Cauliflower, and Potato recipe on page 38 without the added salt.

Wiggly Worm Soup
Make a chicken noodle soup with chicken stock, a little extra finely chopped cooked chicken, broken-up spaghetti, and add some finely chopped vegetables such as broccoli or green onion or a few peas or some corn kernals.

Snail, Star, and Daisy Sandwiches

Sandwiches make a quick snack, light meal, or handy feed-all, for family gatherings and birthday parties. Sure, there's the classic square or triangle cut, but here are a few more ideas to intrigue a young 'un.

Snails
Spread a slice of bread with a sticky filling such as jam, peanut butter, honey (only for children over 12 months) or hummus.

Cut off the crusts (see Witch's Fingernails on page 166 for an idea for what to do with them), then roll the bread up like a jelly roll. Cut across with a sharp knife to reveal the spiral disks and serve on a plate of lettuce leaves.

Stars
Make sandwiches with your chosen fillings then use a star-shaped cookie cutter. Cut-out shapes work well with most other cookie cutters, but remember to choose one that doesn't waste too much.

Daisies
You will need a large flower-shaped cutter and a small round cutter. Cut two bread slices using the flower cutter, then cut out a central hole from just one slice. Spread the flower with a colorful filling (e.g. sliced cheese, ham, jam), then complete the sandwich with the other slice so you can see the filling at the center of the daisy.

Filling ideas
Egg salad (hardboiled egg, mashed with pasteurized mayo).
Grated cheese, grated carrot, diced ham, parsley.
Cream cheese, lemon zest, parsley, and steamed salmon.
Tuna, mayo, corn, lettuce.

Witch's Fingernails

Sounds interesting? Good, because these couldn't be simpler and I have to credit my mom for the exciting name given to what are actually the discarded crusts from party sandwiches (see page 165)!

Crusts cut from slices of bread **1 teaspoon jam**
1 tablespoon butter

Grill the crusts until golden and crunchy. Melt the butter and stir in the jam until runny. Use a pastry brush to paint on the jam "nail polish." Serve on their own, as a purée dipper, or on the side of a main dish or soup. Older children will love painting the Witch's Fingernails themselves, so serve the "polish" in an egg cup.

Real Fruit Ice Pops

Some children go off fruit, maybe because it seems boring compared to all the other sweet things available. Commercial ice pops are typically riddled with synthetic colors and flavors; organic fruit pops are virtually unheard of. To make your own, most recipes suggest adding sugar. I've found they can lack flavor without sweetness, but I prefer to use apple juice instead of refined sugar.
Makes 8 pops (you can buy ice pop molds from most department stores or from specialist kitchen supply stores—check the volume of liquid your set needs)

1 cup seasonal fruit purée **1¾ cups apple juice**
  (see stage 1)

Combine the purée and apple juice in a blender and blend. Pour into the molds and freeze until solid.

   For super-quick ice pops, use frozen fruit purées or crush in a few cubes of ice, so the mixture is very cold even before they're put in the freezer.

Crispy Cakes

These will bring back memories—they're easy to make and great for a young child who wants to learn how to cook. Add a couple of tiny chocolate eggs to turn into a bird's nest.
Makes 15 cakes

⅓ cup butter **4 cups corn flakes or rice**
2–3 tablespoons corn syrup   **crispies**
½ pound milk or bittersweet **15 paper cupcake cases**
  chocolate

In a large saucepan, melt the butter, then reduce to a low heat. Add the syrup and the chocolate (broken into chunks) and stir until melted. Remove from the heat and stir in the cereal. Spoon into the paper cases and leave to cool.

Funny Face Cookies

This simple recipe is a great way to get children involved in cooking.
Makes about 20

1½ cups self-rising flour **1 small egg**
½ cup granulated sugar **1 tablespoon lemon juice**
1 stick butter or margarine
  (chilled)

Preheat the oven to 350°F. Lightly grease a couple of baking sheets.

   Mix the flour and sugar and grate in the butter or margarine. Use your fingers to rub in until the mixture resembles breadcrumbs. Beat the egg and add, with the lemon juice, to the flour mixture and bring it together with your hands to form a firm dough.

   Sprinkle the work surface with a little more flour and roll out. Use cookie cutters to shape, place on the baking sheets and bake for 10–15 minutes until lightly golden. Leave to cool on a wire rack and store in an airtight tin.

Cupcakes, Fairy Cakes, and Butterfly Cakes

Makes 14–16

BASIC CUPCAKE RECIPE:
1 stick butter or margarine
1 cup granulated sugar
2 medium eggs

1 cup self-rising flour
Paper cupcake cases

Preheat the oven to 375°F and set out the paper cases into cup-cake trays.

Cream the butter and sugar until pale in color and creamy in texture. Beat in the eggs one at a time then fold in the flour (sift first if there are any lumps). Half-fill each paper cupcake case and bake for about 20 minutes until firm (check they are cooked through by inserting a metal skewer into one of the cupcakes—if it comes out clean they're ready). Allow to cool. If you plan to freeze them do so at this point, before decorating. For decorating ideas, see below and right.

Butterfly cakes

Decorates 14–16 cupcakes

14–16 cupcakes (see recipe above)
FOR BUTTERFLY CAKE DECORATION
1 tablespoon butter or margarine
1/2 cup confectioners' sugar

Choose flavors from:
2 chunks melted chocolate
1 teaspoon cocoa (adding a little milk if too dry)
2–3 drops vanilla extract
1 teaspoon orange or lemon juice

Cream the butter and confectioners' sugar together—for speed combine using the chopping bowl of a hand blender. Alternatively beat with a fork until pale, smooth, and creamy. Add the chosen flavoring.

To make the butterfly wings, cut a slice from the top of each cake and cut in half. Place a blob of icing in the center of cake top and arrange the wings at angles on top.

Decorating fairy cakes

For speed you can get on with frosting these yourself; for fun involve your child in baking and decorating. It'll be messy and their idea of stylish will probably resemble modern art.

Decorates 14–16 cup cakes

14–16 cupcakes (see recipe left)
TO DECORATE
2 tablespoons confectioners' sugar
2–3 teaspoons water or fruit juice

Natural food coloring (optional), found in specialist organic shops and some supermarkets
Selection of colorful dried fruit, naturally colored cake sprinkles or small chocolate shapes

Sift the icing sugar and gradually stir in the water or juice until smooth and runny enough to be drizzled from a teaspoon. Add the optional food colorings. If using dried fruits cut into sprinkle-sized pieces.

Drizzle the icing on to each cake and decorate.

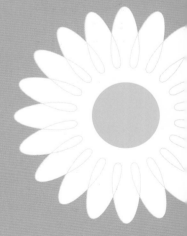

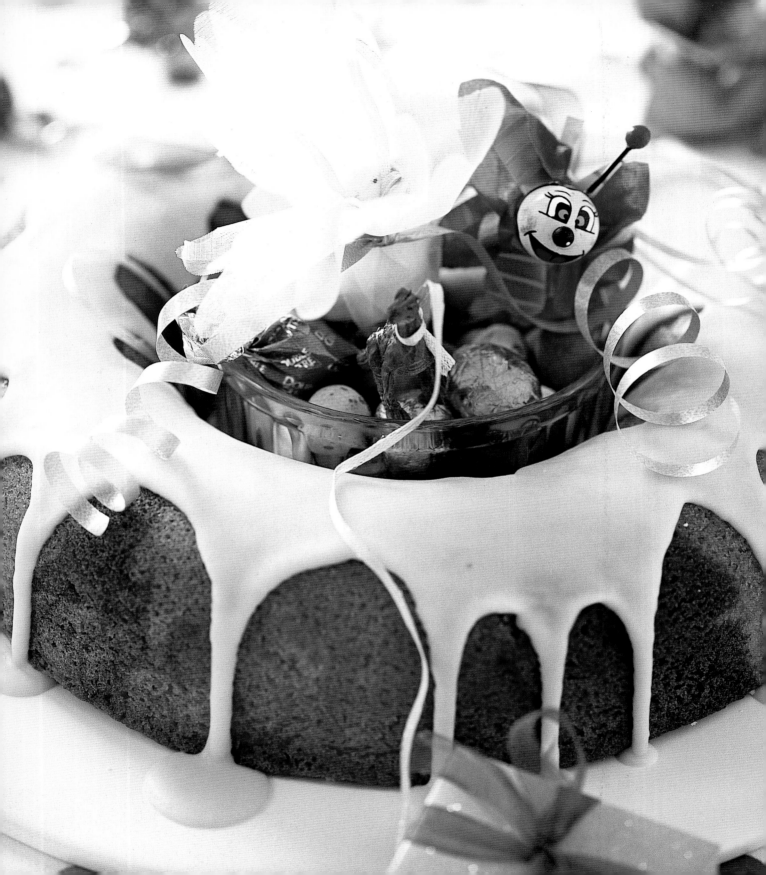

Birthday Surprise Cake

This quick-to-make cake will delight children of all ages and adults too. Simply vary the surprises at the end of the streamers to suit the age of the guests.

Makes 16 child or 8 adult portions
(suitable for freezing before you decorate)

BASIC CAKE MIX
1 cup granulated sugar
2 sticks butter or margarine
(check it is suitable for baking)
4 medium eggs
3 cups self-rising flour
2 tablespoons milk (or orange juice if avoiding milk)
2 tablespoons butter or margarine to grease the cake ring

FOR THE CHOCOLATE MARBLE
1 rounded tablespoon cocoa

FOR THE PALE MARBLE
3–4 drops vanilla extract or grated rind (zest) of 1 unwaxed lemon or orange

FOR THE SURPRISES
Small gift for each guest wrapped in colored paper with a streamer attached

FOR THE FROSTING
1½ cups confectioners' sugar
1 tablespoon warm water or orange juice (adding more as needed)

Preheat the oven to 350°F. Use the extra butter or margarine to grease the inside of a nonstick 10 inch cake mold.

Fast method

Measure the basic ingredients into the bowl of a food processor and beat with the plastic blade until smooth and creamy (2–3 minutes). Spoon out half into a mixing bowl and add the cocoa and beat for another minute (adding a little more milk if needed). Add the vanilla or citrus rind to the remaining mixture.

Traditional method

Combine the sugar and butter, beat with a fork until pale and creamy. Beat the eggs and slowly add. Sift the flour into the mixture, adding the milk as needed to make a smooth, stiff creamy mix. Scoop half into a separate mixing bowl and continue as above.

Using a tablespoon, place spoonfuls of each mixture alternately into the mold until all the mixture has been used. Drag the spoon once through the cake mixture to create the marble effect (don't be tempted to stir further; you will end up with one color rather than two!).

Bake for 30–35 minutes until well risen. To check it is cooked, insert a skewer into the mixture—it should come out clean.

Leave to cool a little, then tap round the mold before turning out on a wire cooling rack.

Make the frosting and use a wet palette knife to smooth over the cake.

Decorate as desired.

Directory

General advice on parenting

Mothering: The Magazine of Natural Family Living
www.mothering.com

www.parenthood.com

www.ivillage.com (link for Pregnancy and Parenting)

Mumsnet
www.mumsnet.com

Guidance on Food Safety and Nutrition

Center for Food Safety and Applied Nutrition
5100 Paint Branch Parkway
College Park, MD 20740-3835
www.cfsan.fda.gov

For Dietary guidelines:
www.healthierus.gov

US Food and Drug Administration (FDA)
5600 Fishers Lane
Rockville, MD 20857-0001
www.fda.gov

Breastfeeding advice

Babies and Moms Peninsula Breastfeeding Center
329 Primrose Ave, Suite 103
Burlingame, CA 94010
www.babiesandmoms.com

For midwives, pregnancy and for parenting and products
www.midwivesonline.com

La Leche League
(For parents in US and Canada)
1400 N. Meacham Road
Schaumburg, IL 60173-4808
Tel: (847) 519-7730
www.lalecheleague.org

The Baby Friendly Initiative
This is a global program of UNICEF and the World Health Organization that works with the health services to improve practice so that parents are enabled and supported to make informed choices about how they feed and care for their babies.
www.babyfriendlyusa.org

Advice for vegetarian and vegan parents

American Vegan Society
56 Dinshah Lane
PO Box 369
Malaga, NJ 08328
www.americanvegan.org

The Vegetarian Resource Group
PO Box 1463
Baltimore, MD 21203
(410) 366 8343
www.vrg.org

Allergies and intolerances

Allergy Prevention Center
1072 Casitas Pass Road
Suite 190
Carpinteria, CA 93013
www.allergypreventioncenter.com

American Dietetic Association
120 South Riverside Plaza
Suite 2000,
Chicago, IL 60606–6995
www.eatright.org

Asthma and Allergy Foundation of America
Deepdene House
1233 20th Street NW
Suite 402
Washington, DC 20036
www.aafa.org

Food Allergy and Anaphylaxis Network
11781 Lee Jackson Highway
Suite 160
Fairfax, VA 22033
www.foodallergy.org

National Resource Center on AD/HD
CHADD
8181 Professional Place
Suite 150,
Landover, MD 20785
www.help4adhd.org

Food and dairy intolerance

International Food Information Council (IFIC)
1100 Connecticut Avenue NW
Suite 430
Washington, DC 20036
Tel: (202) 296 6540
www.ific.org

Gluten intolerance

Celiac.com
www.celiac.com

When to wean

The US Department of Health and Human Services
Richmond House
200 Independence
Avenue S.W
Washington, DC 20201
Tel: (202) 619 0257
Toll free: 1-877-696-6775
www.os.dhhs.gov

World Health Organization
The United Nations
(specialized agency for health)
www.who.int

Research into weaning and food preference development

Monell Chemical Senses Institute
Monell Chemical Senses
Center
3500 Market Street
Philadelphia, PA 19104-3308
www.monell.org
Tel: +44 (215) 898-6666

University Of Birmingham
Dr. Gillian Harris
Department of Applied
Developmental Psychology
The University of
Birmingham
Edgbaston, Birmingham
B15 2TT
Tel: +44 (0121) 414 3344

For more information on organic food

Demeter Association Inc
25844 Butler Road
Junction City, OR 97448
www.demeter-usa.org

Organic Consumers Association
6101 Cliff Estate Road
Little Marrais, MN 55614
www.organicconsumers.org

Organic Trade Association
PO Box 547
Greenfield, MA 01302
www.ota.com

Fresh Daisy
Kinetic House
Theobald Street
Elstree, Herts
WD6 4PJ
Tel: +44 (870) 240 7028
www.daisyfoods.com

Health and safety advisors

The Red Cross
(Offer voluntary advice and information for families and are the world's largest providers of Family First Aid Kits.)
www.redcross.org

www.babycenter.com
The most complete online resource for new and expectant parents.

www.askbaby.com
Everything you need to know about getting pregnant, being pregnant, and parenting.

www.surebaby.com
Information about pregnancy for parents and their babies.

Index

Acknowledgements

Big thanks for all the moms, dads, and babies who inspired this book, for all your questions and shared weaning experiences—the good, bad, and ugly!

Sincere thanks to Ali Hanan, writer, journalist, and mom of Luka, Rosa and big kid Dizzy.

Bruce, thanks for the hard work on the book, dedication to Fresh Daisy and endless support—you make me laugh. Sorry the hip-hop styley reference was cut.

To Alison Fenton, Sandra Lane, Lizzie Harris, Jacqueline Bellefontaine, and Krissy Schmidt—thanks for all your hard work.

Big shout to the mighty Vickster, Mark, Jo, Seb, Quent, Sabine and Peter. Cheers to all at Create, especially head honcho Boyd—maybe VCs aren't so bad.

To Guy – for your vision and positive approach.

To all at Kyle Cathie—especially Muna, for the personable whip cracking and Homer impersonations.

To Green Baby (0870 240 6894/www.greenbaby.co.uk) for the loan of the baby clothes
and
Ezee-Reach Ltd (01908 565001/www.ezee-reach.com) for the springy cutlery on pp.111–112.

Sincere thanks for the expert guidance from Dr. Anita Macdonald, Head of Research Dietetics, Birmingham Children's Hospital.

Finally thanks to supermodels Ben, Zen, Rosa, Rosa, Lily, Amy, Jack, Josh, Harry, and Alice—something for your parents to tease you about when you're 18.

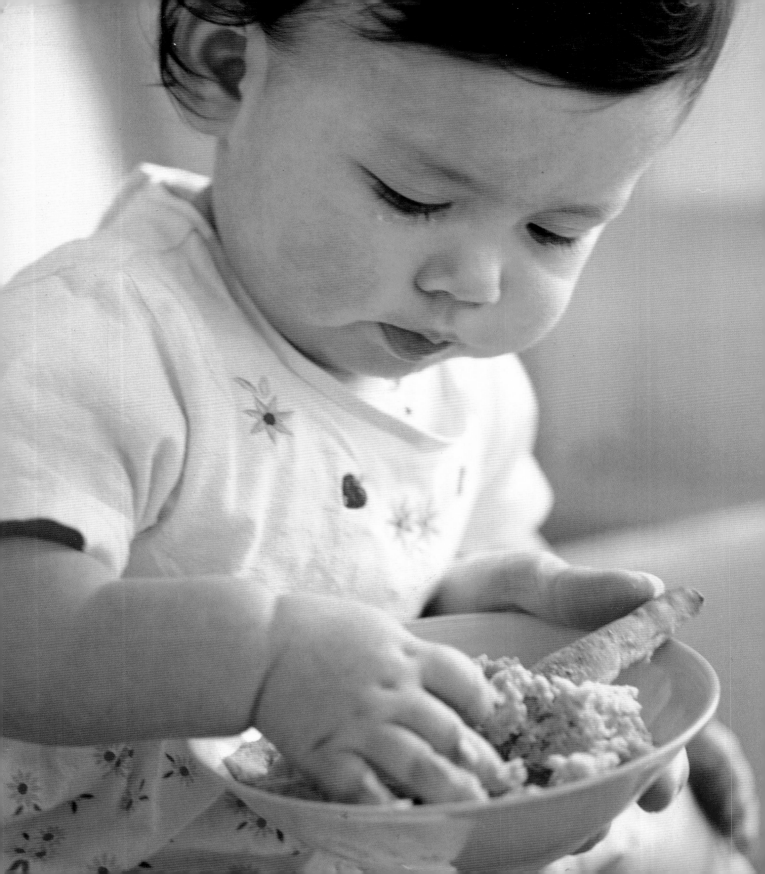